Passion Beyond Pain

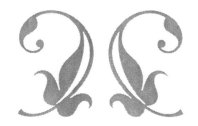

Passion Beyond Pain

A Mindful Approach
to Living a Life of Balance

John Inzerillo, M.D.

Humanics Publishing Group
Atlanta, GA; Lake Worth, FL

Passion Beyond Pain
© 2008 by John Inzerillo, M.D.
a Humanics Publishing Group publication
First Edition

Humanics Publishing Group is a division Brumby Holdings, Inc.

Brumby Holdings, Inc.
12 S. Dixie Highway, Suite 203
Lake Worth, FL 33460
USA
www.humanicspub.com
Phone: 561-533-6231
Fax: 561-533-6233
Email: humanics@mindspring.com

Printed in the United States of America and the United Kingdom

ISBN (Hardcover) 0-89334-453-2
ISBN (Paperback) 0-89334-454-0

Library of Congress Control Number: 200895560

Cover and bookblock design by Marcia Karasoff

Contents

*T*here is a palpable hunger in the world today for health and healing. In seeking to overcome discomfort, pain, and illness the masses are moving toward taking a greater role in making their own health care decisions. With an increasing loss of faith in current day western medicine, even with its incredible technological strides and growing understanding of the mechanisms of disease, many are looking to the east as a new resource for answers. The reality is that the answers have been available for over 2500 years. It is just now that we are beginning to awaken and focus our awareness on the potential to find the places within where we can experience inner and outer health, even in the presence of illness.

Over the past ten to fifteen years there have been a number of health care professionals who have had the wisdom to attempt to incorporate present day knowledge with their growing understanding of ancient medical practices. Like modern day shamans these physicians seek healing for the mind, body, and soul. In the pages of Passion Beyond Pain readers will find insights and practical applications that ease the practitioner into the present moment. Reading and meditating upon the wisdom within these pages one cannot help but experience transformation and thus, greater health. Continuing through the stories readers will find a rekindling of compassion, not only for themselves, but just as important, for others.

In developing a closer connection to the wandering and confusing landscape within, each moment of concentration and practice will allow an opening into the vulnerable places that typically make us feel uncomfortable. With diligent, yet playful practice, a relaxed attitude will supersede all other attitudes and bring greater balance in every aspect of life. Passion Beyond

Pain guides readers gently toward this ever moving goal of balance, to leave them with blossoming evidence that contentment on a daily basis is truly possible. This is not an essay on magical thinking but a discourse on the truth and power of the innate capacity to heal within all of us.

As our population ages there will be increasing numbers of individuals who will be confronted with chronic pain conditions, frailty, and the depression associated with these states of being. There is an urgent and ever increasing need to recognize these symptoms and build a medical community that will successfully and ably deal with these issues. Passion Beyond Pain is another brick in the wall that will assist all of us to care for each other to the best of our abilities as our compassion and understanding matures

Rodney Yee

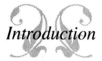

Introduction

THE SPIRITUAL PATH TO HEALTH

*T*he path to wholeness takes many turns. In *Passion Beyond Pain* readers will find ways to create their own sacred space in the process of redefining personal balance and health. By learning to release pain-producing belief systems, new space spontaneously appears. The creative spark, dampened by daily pressures, will once again ignite bringing a sense of ease. In an easy, pressure-free style, wisdom gained from 18 years experience in clinical oncology and 12 years of meditation and yoga practice is shared with readers. With the intention of gaining greater balance in the struggles of life, a mindset has evolved to encompass compassion, caring, patience, and presence. These qualities can be developed and directed not only toward others but also toward the self. The end result is that you lighten up on yourself and find more space for the experiences that truly feed you.

Though suffering is part of life, we were not meant to continually suffer. Anyone experiencing chronic pain conditions such as fibromyalgia, rheumatoid arthritis, osteoarthritis, diabetic neuropathy, or accident related painful injuries knows that pain saps life energy and leaves it's victim empty. These individuals, like myself, feel drained by mid-morning. The goal becomes making it through the rest of the workday, getting home and dealing with the issues there, then trying to get some restful sleep. The problem is that even sleep does not bring relief as pain causes one to toss and turn in an attempt to find a restful position. Waking up fatigued the next morning, the cycle continues.

Living with chronic pain leads to long-term depression. The associated feelings of worthlessness and dread substantiate these feeling as if to mock life. Medication only goes so far in giving any relief. How many ibuprofen can an individual take on a daily basis before an ulcer develops? The side effects of antidepressants take away one's libido and seem to cloud consciousness. Most of our energy goes into trying to tolerate our pain and getting on with life, but there is no room for joy or contentment.

In *Passion Beyond Pain* those suffering from chronic pain conditions, experiencing emotional turmoil, whatever its causes and those living in a state of confusion and wanting to take action to ease their distress will find direction and solace within these pages. Any worthwhile journey takes preparation. The techniques demonstrated in this book prepare the reader for the difficult path ahead. Yes, it seems easier to continue to live as we have been, but that negates any hope for true and lasting joy. We can continue wallowing in old belief systems and pass these beliefs onto our children so that they experience suffering also, or we can make a commitment to ourselves and our families that we will get to the root of our distress and take on new and healthier attitudes.

Passion Beyond Pain is not intended for the weak at heart. It takes tremendous courage to begin looking at our own issues. To decide to take steps to learn about and understand our pain might be equated with taking a stroll through Dante's seven layers of Hell. If we were to wake up this moment and feel the pain that we are running from, we would find that we have been dwelling there for quite some time.

The chapters within will show readers how to first quiet their minds, settle their bodies, then follow the threads of memory that have led to current conditions. The steps to the cultivation of awareness and mindfulness will be described through the following pathways:

☯ Instruction on beginning then progressing with a daily meditation practice (five to ten minutes a day is enough to begin)

☯ Techniques for using the breath to remain in the moment are presented (as long as we are alive our breath is the one constant)

☯ Beginning from a quiet center, light is shed on methods for unlocking frozen energy long repressed in painful memories

☯ Making a reassessment of priorities by generating individually specific questions concerning desires, motivations, and needs

☯ An in-depth study of the ancient *chakra* system (energy centers), with understanding its uses mind-body balance is regained

☯ Chakra manipulation as preventative medicine and stress reduction

☯ Methods for using the breath to massage tight and tired muscles

☯ Using simple yoga postures to focus on healthy attitudes such as love, hope, joy, peace, compassion, and kindness (if you can breathe, you can do yoga)

☯ Instructional meditations for overcoming old habits and addictions, including ways to recognize when others are beginning to push your buttons

☯ Effective non-threatening ways for expressing your needs to those in your circles

☯ How to foster and maintain healthy relationships and support systems especially during times of transition

Passion Beyond Pain is the first book for everyone who suffers from pain. Many times in my practice individuals come in for follow-up and tell me that they can't do anything. They have to get around in wheelchairs because their leg strength is less than optimal or their neck hurts because of years of unrecognized tension. The common thread for all of us is that we have to begin with and work with what we have. If the only thing you can do is lift your leg two inches off the floor then that is what you start doing.

5

This book will show you how to drop the limiting beliefs that are holding you back and start moving toward a life of involvement. The meditations within give readers insight into all of the forces that keep us where we are, but more importantly the energies that move us forward and bring life to our being will be revealed.

Get ready to move into the moment and experience the power of what you have been given right now. The gifts of your own life are awaiting your presence. Turn the page and walk into a refreshing and new consciousness.

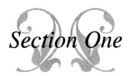

Section One

TOUCHING THE PAST

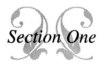

Section One

TOUCHING THE PAST

Introduction

*W*e are inexorably connected to past events in our lives. There is only one way to free us from this bondage and that is by intentionally bringing ourselves back to the present moment, every moment. In our attempts to remain aware we, with practice, can begin to notice more quickly when we have left the present. This takes willingness fostered by diligence, and is achievable to everyone. The pace becomes your choice depending on your courage and willingness to stay focused and in the moment.

Without the habitual responses attributable to memory we stand helpless, in a sorry state, relearning even the simplest tasks. Without memory we would fail to make any progress as a society. The dark, paralyzing, side of memory comes into play when we allow repressed fear responses to keep us stuck. With its resultant frustration and confusion this memory lock serves no useful purpose. It is possible to stay in the present and yet consciously review past events with an objective eye. This practice first has to be cultivated by desire in action.

The emotional charge sealed within a memory is what we are looking to release. Over the years an immeasurable quantity of pain, anger, and fear can accumulate and result in chronic pain. This is pain whose etiology is undetected by CAT scans, MRI's and blood work. The only telltale signs on X-rays might be varying degrees of degenerative changes in the bones due to constant muscle tension. The sad part of this is we are unaware of the fact that we do this to ourselves. To reverse the process we must wake up.

We all have our own personal stories and memories of closeness with those we love. There are also the self-induced fear responses that have formed and piled up over the years that stop us from looking deeper into our desires and moving closer our true selves. We have learned through fear how to tighten-up, squeeze down, and lock our energy into muscle tissue. As we age there is a gradual thawing of this frozen energy and unless we look at these issues with a clear eye we will experience greater physical pain over time. Our painful memories can haunt us as we continue our attempts to ignore them or they can be the power behind our healing, if we are willing to do the work required.

After completing my oncology training, one of my first cancer patients was a middle-aged woman who developed breast cancer. Luckily it was an early stage cancer, but it was a large enough tumor to require a mastectomy. She opted to have the surgery followed by chemotherapy and decided to have a delayed breast reconstruction after completing her primary therapy.

I recall stopping in to see her the morning after her surgery. She was having tremendous post-operative pain and all I could do was recommend giving more pain medicine. Her chest was packed with heavy bandages and there were Jackson-Pratt drains, half-filled with serosanguineous fluid, sticking out of her body, surrounding the surgical site. Wheeled IV poles that held and infused normal saline, antibiotics, and morphine surrounded the head of her bed.

I can only look back now and wish I could tell her what I know today about dealing with pain and our daily challenges. Over the past 10 years I have undertaken the study and practice of meditation and yoga. I needed, as we all do, a way to find balance in the midst of a hectic medical practice, where I was dealing with death and dying all of the time. With such a busy practice it was easy to ignore the needs of my young family or worse come home and be tired and cranky.

Yoga and meditation became my anchor as it has recently for my patient described above. I see her just about every week now, but not for medical follow-up or cancer surveillance. She also suffers from fibromyalgia, with its migratory arthritic pains and trigger points. In an effort to cope with and ease some of the associated pain and discomfort she continually experiences, she comes to our weekly yoga class that I instruct at the office. Along with three or four, and sometimes five or six, other folks we spend an hour and a half a week taking care of ourselves by working with our breath, mind, and muscles. In the course of a few months I have noticed a definite improvement in her flexibility and greater confidence in her performance of the asanas or postures.

It is key to begin our journey from a safe place. Unfortunately most of us do not feel safe when it comes to past events that continue to bother us and we would rather smoke a cigarette, have a beer, do the dishes, waste away the hours on the internet, or just take a nap to avoid our pain. Yoga and meditation offer us this safe haven.

We all have experienced stressful events in relation to family matters. Each of us knows the pain associated with the loss of a loved one. Unresolved issues are especially troublesome and may cause distress for years unless there is a conscious decision to crack open that box of tangled emotions, beliefs and attitudes. Seeing a family member through a difficult and complicated medical illness can be a wellspring of wisdom. Certainly no one feels that way while the minute to minute, sometimes critical, events are unfolding day by day, but many times after the acute event has resolved there is time to let the high energy charge subside. This opens up space for an objective evaluation of feelings and emotions. It becomes a time of priority redistribution or in some cases an opportunity to initiate the first steps in developing priorities. With this time comes a reevaluation of motives and a hard look at what is truly meaningful in your life. The stressful family event takes us out of the cycle of daily routines and takes our minds off of the usual obsessions of our minds. Such an event acts as the sledgehammer that makes the first crack in our internal concrete thinking. We think we know it all and have everything figured out, then WHACK! a family member gets sick and life as we know it ends. It can be the first indication that there is hope for growth and change.

We all know someone who has been through such difficult times that we wonder how they ever saw it through to the end and were able to remain productive and civil. There is such an individual in our community who has been through the fire over a family medical tragedy. She married young, became pregnant and gave birth to a healthy son who is my son's peer. After a few years she had a second son who was born the picture of health. One day he became ill, had a seizure and was never the same. He became dependent on a ventilator, requiring twenty-four hour care which fortunately was given in his home. This young mother grew up quickly and did everything she could to improve the quality of her son's life. In all of the pain she experienced, she remained outgoing and friendly and continued to invest the majority of her energies into caring for her loved ones. Eventually her weakened child died of progressive respiratory problems. Instead of falling into depression and despair she decided to go back to school. She now serves caring for the sick as a licensed practical nurse. She was fortunate in that she was able to take her grief and pain and channel it almost immediately into something positive for herself, her family, and her community.

It is unfortunate that we are not all able to take such painful events and life histories and transform them into such healing stories. Many of us are thrust into painful situations and are ill equipped to deal with the emotional stress to follow. The seeds of anger, disappointment, resentment, and fear are planted and we reap the sins of chronic depression, unrelenting and nagging pain, and go around feeling that life has passed us by.

To allow ourselves to process such painful events we have to enable ourselves to dwell in the place of uncertainly. We still remain responsible for the general direction of our lives, but when we allow ourselves to entertain the idea of uncertainty, we do not have to worry about all of the details. This knowledge is liberating. We do not have to start out knowing all of the answers. It is so much easier to realize that to relax and let our individual stories unfold is the natural way to health and balance.

Chapter One

Awakening Through Memories: The Power of Recall

*U*nlike footprints in the sand, past experiences are stored in microscopic electrical relay stations in the brain, called neurons and remain there for the rest of our lives. The complex signaling that transpires between each individual neuron and its multitude of connections occurs at the speed of light. The release and subsequent uptake of neurotransmitters moving across a synapse travel much like a ferryboat carrying cars and passengers across a bay. These are the things that memories are made of. Much of past experience resides below the surface of awareness but continually dictates perception as well as action. Images rise into consciousness like floating; ever-changing clouds, then fade as quickly as a popping bubble.

Locking onto a single memory and consciously dwelling there leads to stagnation and inhibition of the natural flow of energy or life force. What we choose to recall and why remains a mystery, but the interconnection and play of emotions, feelings, attitudes, and temperament come together to construct precisely what we are and from these interactions our memories congeal.

Our use of memory goes beyond our aptitude to remember a list of spelling words or reciting the multiplication tables. We can use our memories to relive emotions evoked through touching and thought provoking poems and verse; verse that may stay with us and add flavor to everything we do from that moment on. Memory also serves to help us make complex decisions and helps us plan and manage our time. It allows us to communicate effectively and shows us how to be more creative. As an instrument of our potential, our memory works like a slave to bring greater imagination into our problem solving.

We approach everything from our own perspective. All of our decisions and our preconceived outcomes are dictated by past experience. Through the use of meditation we come to a place where we begin to broaden our perspectives. Our meditation may result in insights through a technique described by Michael Morgan in his book, *Creating Workforce Innovation: Turning Individual Creativity into Organizational Innovation.* Here he describes the use of a Reframing Matrix in which the readers are shown ways of looking at problems with a different perspective.

Meditation, or sitting in silence, brings us to a place where we see all sides of an issue with greater clarity. As we continue in our practice, instead of being pulled in one direction by a dominant idea, all thoughts are given equal attention so that the most appropriate choice will eventually manifest for us.

There is no way around it, we all have problems and will continue to have problems. It is our attitude toward these problems and our confidence in solving the problems that is paramount. Most individuals come to meditation because of an overwhelming sense of confusion over their problems or unresolved issues. Looking for a way to come to grips with our presumed deficiencies some of us fall into meditation, others use yoga or both, while others run, swim, hike, or bike. There appears to be some need to be better, stronger, faster, and quicker of mind than we are. Somewhere in our memory banks there are the black clouds of insufficiency, impotence in the face of challenges, and a general sense of unease.

In the Reframing Matrix, Michael Morgan describes the 4 "P" approach in which first we look at the "Product perspective." In this paradigm we are the products. We were given individual talents and it is our work to learn to express these gifts to the best of our ability. When we doubt that we are in possession of such gifts we plant the seeds of discontent. Our life goal then becomes moving in the direction of self-acceptance and coming to a place where we are able to acknowledge these special gifts.

The remaining aspects of his work include an examination of a "Planning perspective," followed by an evaluation of the "Potential perspective", and finally the "People perspective." In the multitude of things that we chose to do with our lives, we seem to start off with the perspective that there is something wrong with us (the Product perspective). We need to come to a place where we can safely question if there is something about our modus operandi that is at fault (the Planning perspective). Once we have summoned the courage to ask that question then the query begins on how to achieve what we want. For most of us we may want to be more comfortable in our own skin no matter what is going on around us (the Potential perspective). Finally with the People perspective we look for ways to relate to others in more satisfying ways.

By tending to our memories we automatically begin to question if what we have been doing is what we need to continue to do to achieve a desired result. We may find that it is time to drop old patterns of thinking and look for new ways of seeing. Sitting with ourselves is a surefire way to break down the barriers that have led to the lockdown of memory and the closing of potential energy sources. Like the Chicago Police Department, our memories serve to protect. It is such protection that keeps us in our comfortable, safe, yet smelly and isolated cocoon.

Institutions such as McDonald's, Hardee's, Burger King, and Wendy's continue to flourish and operate in the black as they have done for years. The CEO's of these American eateries are banking on the continued use of memory by the average consumer. By today's numbers, 60% of the adult American population suffers from obesity. This translates into about 127 million people, and the numbers are on the rise. Obesity contributes to the development of cancers of the breast, prostate, and colon. Combining these conditions with its contribution to heart disease, diabetes, high blood pressure, and stroke, there are 300,000 excess deaths per year in the U.S. due to the ravages of obesity. Even though obesity is a chronic disease with a strong familial component, its ability to persist and prevail in society is due to an environment which does not stress or reward physical activity and which has an overabundance of high-calorie, low cost foods. Meditation and yoga will help us break the bonds of the addictions that keep us overeating and that keep our sense of self-esteem in the basement. In a mindful state we will make healthier dietary choices and our physical and mental well being will benefit.

There appears to be a consensus in psychology today that temperaments such as hopefulness and optimism and their counterparts hopelessness and pessimism seem to be personality traits which have predominantly a genetic basis with environmental factors contributing to an unknown degree as a child develops. Today there are websites offering free personalized temperament descriptions with the promise of showing us ways to harness the power of personality. These sites spell out how we can build stronger relationships by improving communication and interpersonal skills.

We are shown how easy it can be to meet others' expectations by better understanding people's styles, and how to diffuse interpersonal problems by gaining sensitivity to others' perspectives. The final promise will have us achieving valuable self-knowledge into core motivations and attaining personal and professional goals by learning to capitalize on strengths. This is all well and good and these concepts and facts are useful to know but they all lack the power of heart and soul insight that is available with a daily meditation practice. In such a practice it becomes you with your thoughts. As long as you remain gentle with yourself you will be able to sit with many of the issues that come up and gain new insights into what forces move you. With time you will be able to determine why you believe what you believe. This knowledge becomes the fuel for change in the direction that you need to go.

It is one thing to be told how to go about achieving something and it is another to experience these events first hand. The psychological path is geared to change that which we and others have decided is not useful in a goal oriented society whereas meditation is a tool that can be employed to help us become more comfortable with what is, thus allowing transformation to occur individually and naturally from within. From this perspective even memories that are holding us back and have us spinning our wheels like Big Daddy Don Garlits would in his AA fuel-injected dragster on the ice of Lake Michigan, in the middle of February, can be viewed as grist for the mill. If given permission and if we proceed with a kind heart we can make use of all of our past experience, especially the rough and tough times. With the fostering of awareness we can choose where our dominant thoughts reside regardless of our genetically determined temperaments.

It is natural to want to cling to happy and joyous memories but when it comes to repressing these less than memorable images we expend energy. This energy expenditure removes us from the pleasures of the moment. Instead of living in the flow of natural energy, we choose to resist painful memories and thus end up exhausted. Such ways of operating lead to chronic fatigue, depression, and an absence of zest in our lives.

Every six months I see a young female patient for follow-up. We originally met when I was consulted to evaluate her for a blood clotting disorder. She has an abnormal protein in her blood that is called an antiphospholipid antibody. The presence of this antibody is the least of her problems as she suffers from obesity, hypertension, major depression, fibromyalgia, and temperomandibular joint dysfunction. She has to wear a tooth guard 24 hours a day to help relieve the pain in her jaw.

To complicate things her husband is well-trained in computers but has been unable to secure appropriate work for his training. Though she looks and lives the picture of misery, she continues to truck on. She has channeled her limited energies into the formation of a Fibromyalgia Support Group that meet once a month at the local YMCA, and has recently embarked on a training program that will allow her to do counseling. We have worked together, to a limited degree, with breath work to help release some of her chronic muscle tension.

While we are in a relaxed mode, memories seem to dance, prance, and wander into our minds. Majestically directed by each outside stimulus, be it the scent of freshly cut grass in the spring or the sound of the rapping beak of a woodpecker digging into breakfast on a nearby oak, our minds move effortlessly with these natural events. In the absence of inner conflict there is no resistance to what is. It is when we are uptight and tense that these same memories come at us like jumbled messages received by a CIA satellite. In such a state we have a limited capacity to separate out these images and we end up confused.

17

Developing awareness of these functions of the mind is the first step to making more space within and allows for greater understanding of our role in the entire process.

With this said, may we all open enough and gently begin to do as Pema Chodron, a Buddhist nun who has written extensively on the subject of meditation, has instructed. She has written as part of her concluding aspiration in *The Places That Scare You, A Guide to Fearlessness in Difficult Times*, "May we clearly see all the barriers we erect between ourselves and others to be as insubstantial as our dreams," and "May we go to the places that scare us."

For the philosopher, recollective memory is the episodic memory of modern day psychology. This is also known as personal memory or direct memory. This is the memory that floods into consciousness when a middle-aged daughter realizes her father's death is eminent. She brings her eighty-eight year old dad into the office because he's had a prior stroke and his heart is plumb worn out from beating too many times against the supernormal resistance in his vessels created by longstanding high blood pressure. As a consequence of both disorders, he is so weak that he can't brush his own teeth or put on his own socks.

This day she realizes that modern medicine can do no more for her greatest love and comes face to face with the mortality of this gift she has held closely since her first memories. In this case, memories flood the mind like a sunami drenching and destroying a seaside village. Those millions of moments with dad, some real, some idealized, some fantasized, but all packed with intense feeling may be the only treasures left after her loss and there will be no further opportunity to create these gems for the soul. She is left with an overwhelming sense of loneliness and loss feeling her only recourse is to shed tears. Why does she apologize for her show of emotion when we have all been there? Every one of us has faced crisis where close family or friends are in danger and we have all been subjected to the realities of loss.

We may question emotionally how could a good God take such a wonderful person from us who has helped us through some of our worst times. The memories of the first bike ride after getting that brand new bicycle for

Christmas, the times you were allowed to take the car to school after getting up early to take dad to work, the pride in your loved one's eyes seeing you graduate or walk down the isle in Holy Matrimony. The tide of emotions peak and the fuse of the mind blows and it is a time for tears. Yet we apologize. It is all right to cry. It is healthy to cry. At least this is the way we would hope that our thinking goes, but in everyday life too many men and some women have the memory of being told that it is a sign of weakness to cry.

Children hear from their moms and dads, "Shut up or I will give you something to cry about." The child may have sustained a physical injury and yet is told that, "It's nothing, don't cry." Why not let a child feel what they know they are feeling? If they are very young and cry it may be that they are crying out of frustration and being in a position of immaturity they simply have no understanding of how to express this human emotion in any other way. Instead the parents get frustrated themselves and can't figure out why Johnny is crying. Let's begin to look beyond the obvious and look into our own memories to see how we were responded to. Then we are able to make a conscious decision based on real-time information and we will have connected with our child. It does not have to be uncomfortable being in the presence of someone who is crying.

If we can allow the tears to flow without wanting to leave the room and stay with that other person in pain, we can ride the tide of emotions and make conditions just so that both of us experience a healing. I don't know where everyone gets the idea that we need to be "healed" like it is a one-time event. What we need and what we can intentionally do for ourselves is to stay open to healing at all times, and experience healing over and over again. The physician who pats a patient or family member on the shoulder and says, "There, there," does not serve the patient nor the self. Crying together makes for connection and healing. Ellen Birx, Ph.D., R.N. has very eloquently expressed the same idea in *Healing Zen: Awakening to a Life of Wholeness and Compassion While Caring for Yourself and Others.* Her words are as follows:

"Healing yourself is also the foundation for healing others. Both the caregiver and the person being cared for can learn and grow with each healing encounter. As you heal both yourself and others will become increasingly aware of the wholeness of life."

Growing up we are many times overcome with such emotion and pain. We find ourselves riding down the hill too fast on that new bike and slam on the brakes only to find that now the rear wheel is flying up over our head and our head is moving quickly toward the ground in front of us. In a flash, as we hit the ground, our breath is knocked and forced from our lungs and for a moment, though it seems like forever, we can't catch our breath. It's only seconds later that we feel the burning, stinging, searing pain radiating from our scraped elbow, knees, and chin. Looking at our injuries we see and then feel the blood. After getting over the initial state of shock and catching those first breaths, we try to move and come to balance. This memory remains and will forever influence the way you ride your bike, drive your car or even take your next step. As John Sutton tells us in *Memory, The Stanford Encyclopedia of Philosophy*, "remembering is often suffused with emotion. It is connected in obscure ways with dreaming. Memory seems to be a source of knowledge, or perhaps just is retained knowledge."

Our memories can make our lives pleasurable and easy or turn our journey into a mere existence. Memories also have the power to make us completely miserable. We can be so wrapped up in painful memories that we end up physically drained expending much of our energy in maintaining defense mechanisms. Awareness of the power of the mind is a crucial step to liberation. It is also a necessary first step to take action to reverse the damage that has been done.

We have all been in ruts, some lasting longer than others have. The freshness that opens up once we begin to pull ourselves from these ruts is renewing. In this first exercise you will be directed to settle the mind and open the senses to experience the energy behind your stuck places. First, it is important to find a quite and comfortable place to sit. The temperature should not be to any extreme. If you are intending to do this in the early morning hours a light blanket or a full-length bathrobe will probably be enough to keep you comfortable. We do not want to distract the mind with being either to hot or too cold. Our intention is to get into a safe place that is conducive to inner exploration.

Once a comfortable place has been established you will find it helpful to sit on a pillow or folded blanket. The pillow should be firm enough to raise you hips at least three to four inches off the floor. This will assist you in sitting on the "sit bones" of the underside of the pelvis. This posture will help bring the natural inward curvature of the lower spine into proper alignment. With the spine in this natural position there will be less muscular pulling of the upper back, shoulders, and neck thus helping the throat and neck release.

In the beginning it may help to place your pillow or folded blanket up against a wall giving your back a source of feedback for alignment from a front to back and side to side perspective.

Sit yourself with the back of the pelvis as close to the wall as possible. If it is easy for you to cross your legs into a simple sitting position then do so. If not, then keep the knees raised by resting them on pillows or blankets. Yoga blocks will also do here. Next, rest your forearms and hands on your thighs with the palms facing up and open. This places your mind and body into a receptive mode thus preparing you for the insights to follow.

Now that you are comfortable, with the eyes either opened or closed, slowly take in three deep belly breaths. Feel the outward movement of the lower abdomi-

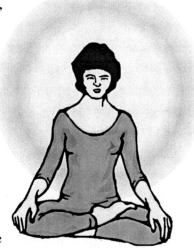

Proper sitting position

nal muscles and the opening stretch of the broadening lower back as the breath begins to bathe your abdominal organs. In the same flowing movement sense the upward creeping oxygen travel toward your upper chest, like ivy snaking its way up a tree trunk as it makes its way toward the sun. In the third part of the breath allow the upper lungs or, the apices, to receive this same purifying inspiration. As the air courses into the uppermost bronchial tubes, or airways, feel the upper back as it moves toward the supporting wall. At the same time allow the shoulders to broaden thus making more space within the upper chest cavity for lung expansion.

As you find the top of the breath consciously calm yourself and resist the urge to struggle. Notice when and where the in-breath stops. Notice the space between the breath. See where the breath begins to move outward and begin emptying the lungs from the apices, then the mid-lungs, and finally allow the inward movement of the muscles of the belly to gently push the residual air up out of the lower lungs. As you do this feel the belly button moving toward the spine. Again resist the urge to tense up and intentionally relax. As you initiate and proceed with the out-breath resist the natural tendency of letting the upper chest collapse. Instead keep the upper chest and shoulders strong against the wall, but not forced. Later in your practice you will find that you can use the out-breath to assist in lengthening the spine even more than you had with the in-breath.

Continue this process for as long as it takes you to center. Now that you have some sense of quiet and inner peace begin to scan your body. This can be done randomly by bringing your gentle attention to each side of the body and comparing muscle tension between the two areas. A problem area for many includes tightness in the shoulders as the position required to work over a keyboard crunches the body in toward the middle and creates constriction of these muscle groups. The source of this muscle contraction is deep and hidden so do not expect to determine its root in one day. Muscle has it's own memory and like a young elephant, it doesn't forget anything.

Muscle is made up of two major proteins known as actin and myosin. Actin is a thin filament and myosin is a thick filament. One thick myosin filament slides over two thin, actin filaments during muscle contraction. Myosin "heads" interact with regions on the actin membrane. These heads have spiny projections that make contact with the actin and bite into it during contraction. Imagine these thorny barbs grabbing onto actin and not releasing because of self-imposed tension. This is the pain chronically felt by those who suffer from conditions such as fibromyalgia. Try squeezing your fist as tight as you can and holding it there. In a few moments it begins to hurt. If you look at the skin on the closed fist there are areas of blanched white skin that are now devoid of blood flow. Others parts of the skin are intensely hyperemic, or red, because of the presence of trapped blood.

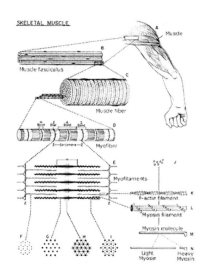

Muscle elements

Now imagine never being able to release the tension in the fist. You will experience chronic pain until the decreased blood flow causes the sensory nerves to deaden. After this there will be only numbness. Muscle contraction is energy dependent in that the body utilizes ATP (adenosine triphosphate, the energy currency of our body) to allow these interactions to occur.

It takes energy, a lot of energy to deal with the stresses of everyday life. Squeezing muscles and holding tension because of emotional trauma leaves us feeling tired and exhausted at the end of the day. When such conditions go unrecognized we have the makings for chronic fatigue, irritability, and over time depression. Unless we consciously allow our muscles to relax after an emotional or physical insult, they will remain in the contracted state thus causing us chronic muscle tension and pain.

In today's society many find it easier to smoke cigarettes, drink alcohol, or use drugs to help get relief from this chronic tension. Unfortunately such reactions to stress do nothing to release the tension at its root. Each muscle has an optimum length at which it contracts and relaxes. Any prolonged contraction or any over-stretching can lead to dysfunction in a particular muscle group. A good example is seen when someone develops congestive heart failure. An individual with chronic hypertension will at first develop a heart that becomes hypertrophied. This simply means that with the increased work that the heart has to perform, because it has to push blood through a circulatory system that has greater resistance, the heart, being a muscle, does what any other muscle will do when it has to work harder. The muscles, in this case the heart, gets bigger. This getting bigger is OK to a degree but when the range for optimal length of the muscle is exceeded then the muscle begins to lose its ability to contract effectively. Thus with each heartbeat, instead of all of the blood and fluids being pumped forward, the back- pressure allows fluid to build up in the lungs and the individual experiences shortness of breath. At first the shortness of breath occurs with exertion and over time and worsening of the congestive heart failure it occurs at rest.

Capillary blood flow will decrease in muscles that are chronically contracted because of stress. For muscles to remain healthy and pain-free they need adequate blood flow. With decreased blood flow the muscle no longer functions optimally and begins to ache. It will remain in this painful state until blood flow is reestablished. Continued stress and reduced blood flow eventually cause the muscle to atrophy. The muscle can become so tight that the individual experiences a contracture and the body takes on a contorted shape. The majority of bad backs are not due to congenital deformities but to what we do to ourselves because of our reaction to stress.

Myofascia is a thin, almost translucent film that wraps around muscle tissue. It's like Saran Wrap or Clingwrap, but for muscles. Each muscle fiber, and some muscle fibers are as short as thirty microns, is covered by myofascia. As muscle fibers come together to form muscle bundles, each muscle bundle is also wrapped in myofascia. Broad bands of fascia help hold muscle fibers together at their origin and insertion points on bones. A good example of this is the fascia that keeps our trapezius muscle, the broad muscle covering our middle and upper back, attached to each spinous process of our vertebral bodies. A similar broad band of fascia is positioned over the lower back that keeps these muscles, bones, ligaments, and tendons in place. As muscle has memory so does myofascia. Hans Selye, "The Father of Stress Theory," brought to us the well-known reaction to stress of "Flight or Fight." When we are stressed we prepare our bodies to either rise to the occasion and fight with all of our ability or we prepare to run. Of course this is a primitive reaction but unless we have consciously worked to look for more effective ways to respond, this is what has been built into the system, and this is how we will respond.

Repeated stressors cause what is referred to as calciphylaxis, or an induced hypersensitivity in which tissues respond to stress with a sudden calcification. One can see how this happens since muscle not only uses ATP for contraction but also uses calcium, sodium, potassium and other co-factors for function. The action potential that occurs when a nerve fires is actually the movement of sodium and potassium across the nerve membrane. With thickening and loss of elasticity, neurotransmitters like epinephrine, acetylcholine, and serotonin, lose their ability to keep communication open between the mind and the body. Tight fascia can not only constrict blood vessels but it can also entrap nerves and eventually form adhesions and scar tissue. So when someone says they were scarred by a psychological or an emotional event they are speaking the truth. Calcium is like stone and when muscle fascia develops calcifications it becomes rock-hard, limiting mobility and thus causing pain.

Over time with the chronic entrapment of nerve bundles, neuropraxia will develop. Neuropraxia is the loss of nerve conduction causing aching pains, numbness, tingling, and hypersensitivity. This condition is best exemplified in those with fibromyalgia but is also well demonstrated in those suffering from TMJ or temperomandibular joint dysfunction, with the chronic tightness, numbness, pain, and ache.

Muscles are meant to help us function optimally. When we ache and hurt we can step back and ask what our role is in the causation and maintenance of this pain. We are the ones who allow the stressors to build up and take their toll on our muscles. The muscles are only doing what we allow them to do. A great example of what a muscle should do normally and what it can do over time if we continue to go through life unaware, is the function of the erector spinae muscle of the back. These thick tubular muscle bundles are also known as the paraspinal muscles. They run along both sides of the spine where they can be easily felt. The contracted or normal state of these muscles keeps our backs erect.

How many times as a kid were you told to sit up straight? In school overwhelmed with work, tired of sitting at a desk for six hours a day, we slouched to take a break, to escape. Not knowing that repositioning, sitting up straight, and taking some deep breaths into the full length of our spines would reenergize us, we continued slouching. This unnatural position was held until recess. Running and breathing deeply, jumping and bending backwards to greet the mid-morning sun, the warmth and fresh air melted away the poisons of stagnation. With freedom of movement and the excitement of the crowd of other children we found ourselves energized once again. No wonder we like vacations and find it hard to transition back to work after a break.

With accumulated hurt we also learned to cover or protect our hearts. In response to the pain we decided to shield our hearts and not leave them open to more pain. This will be explained in greater detail in the discussion about *chakras* in a later chapter. Bending the upper body, folding it over our hearts, effectively closes the door to feeling more pain. It also opposes and antagonizes the normal action of the erector spinae muscles so they become over-stretched and with time, achy and painful. We end up with chronic back pain. Everyone knows how some elderly folks walk with their canes, bent over, afraid of falling. They have chosen to protect their hearts from further injury, as it was all that they knew. Sure it kept a lot of good out but it didn't let anymore bad in.

The erector spinae, when allowed to function normally, will allow for the normal lumbar curve of the lower spine. When the teacher or your mom said sit up straight they did not mean to sit up straight like a board. There is an imaginary line of energy that runs up the front portion of the vertebral bodies. It is that line of energy that needs to be straight to run energy without blockage. Remember how your lower back felt while you were sitting up against the wall during the first meditation exercise? This is how our low back should always be held.

We have to imagine our individual vertebral bodies as if they are building blocks like circular Legos but with little bony projections coming off the sides and back. In between each vertebral body there is a spongy, gelatinous material known as the nucleus propulsus. These are the discs that slip when someone says they have a slipped disc. When we stand or sit out of our natural alignment the discs are allowed to compress upon themselves. With this chronic stimulus they begin to harden and lose their water content. They desiccate or dry out and become brittle and fragile. This process also allows them to more easily slip out of place, resulting in back pain and sometimes radiation of that pain down into the hips and legs.

It is imperative that we take the time to learn about and direct our own energy. If we are not willing to take responsibility for our own energy no one else will and we will suffer. Unprocessed emotions and feelings have the power to keep us down. They are the chains that bind our ability to enjoy. Repressing such feeling does not come without cost. We pay the price of pain, irritability, fatigue, anxiety, and a sense of persistent hopelessness.

One way to help these painful emotions surface, where we are able to start to objectively look at them, is through letter writing. In the process of writing we find there will be more to work with during our meditation sessions. Painful issues can be overwhelming, so it is recommended that with letter writing your intention should be to gather insight and do no harm to self or others. With this said, writing will give you a safer place to express your feelings than a one on one, personal confrontation will. You will also find writing letters to deceased parents can diffuse and untangle your emotions.

Even in the ideal family there will be issues between mothers and daughters and fathers and sons that will continue to be a source of discomfort in the relationships. By making the conscious decision to explore some of these issues you have taken the first steps toward developing greater compassion for yourself and others.

There are definite connections between writing and healing. Even in extreme cases such as those suffering from terminal renal cell carcinoma (kidney cancer) it was found that those individuals who wrote about their feelings concerning their cancer experienced improved quality of sleep, less interruptions of sleep, greater length of their sleep cycle, and less dysfunction during waking hours.

In your daily writing you are free to express any and all issues. In writing down your memories, fears, doubts, and concerns you will also find that emotions such as joy, thankfulness, and even satisfaction and contentment will eventually begin to surface. In putting your ideas on paper you become the creator of your own healing process. You can redo events of the past by injecting your hoped for result. Writing it down makes it real for you.

In writing your letter to Mom or Dad, or for that matter anyone with whom you are having difficulty, feel free to express your emotions no matter how intense. It helps to ground yourself with the earth and use your abdominal breathing techniques once you get on a roll with emotional expression. As you feel your writing hand tense or your jaw muscles clench, imagine a conduit of energy connecting your lower pelvis with the core of the earth. Then consciously allow your jaw to repetitively open and close then move side to side to further manipulate the frozen energy that has been trapped in these muscles because of your emotional history.

Here no one will attack you or tell you that you are wrong. Here you have total control, yet you will find as you continue to write you voluntarily let go of the need to control. You begin to find that you are developing a greater presence with yourself and what the other person thought is only incidental.

Pour your guts out. Take a break if you have to then come back to the writing daily, even if for ten minutes. Memories that have been long forgotten and repressed will begin to surface. Now the task becomes looking even closer at these thoughts, ideas, and beliefs from the safety of your meditation posture.

Go to your quiet place, center yourself with your breathing then follow the images and scenes that arise. You may find your mind takes you to the same scene many days in a row. When this happens gently ask yourself what you were feeling at that time in your life? What significant life events were happening for you and what was changing in your family life? There is no need to force any issue. Simply breathe easily, stay grounded, observe, and gently ask what you need to ask. Your memory wants to serve you. Help it bring your needs to light by staying present and attentive. When fear arises ask yourself if you can stay with it a while longer, as it will pass. If you need to take a break, do so and try again tomorrow.

Chapter Two

Whose Timetable Are You On?

*T*ime and memory have a way of working together. We perform a task, it takes a certain amount of time to complete, and we have the potential to remember every aspect about the performance of that task. It seems that memory is a storage place for time, but reflecting upon the concept of time in our day to day activities, we come to the conclusion that time is man-made. It has become a measuring stick for when we have to go to work, when we get off, when we have to pick up the kids from school, and even when it's time to bake another birthday cake.

In today's world, time is equivalent to pressure. It is such a pleasure when someone tells me to take my time and they really mean it. How many times in the past week have you told yourself to slow down and enjoy the moment? If not more than seven then you have a lot of room to make time for yourself. The majority of our time pressures are self-induced. We push the snooze button on the alarm five times before getting up, wait until the last minute to finish the report that's due in the morning, spend more time planning our summer vacation than we do planning the day in front of us. Most of us think lists make us appear forgetful or semi-senile, so we don't use them, but if we start making daily lists the chances are greater that we will get more done in less time.

By recognizing that time is a tool we begin to lessen the grip that time and clocks have on our psyche. With our highly developed human minds we are completely aware that our time on this earth is limited. This knowledge in itself puts a lot of pressure on us to get the things done that we think we need to do to make us feel that our lives are worthwhile. If we find that we have fallen away from our self-prescribed schedule, frustration knocks on our door louder and louder every day and time becomes the enemy.

Even though we know better, many of us live our days thinking we have all the time in the world. We are under the weight of the clock and our days are numbered, but when we procrastinate we are effectively saying that time and our energy are unimportant to us. When we delay taking the time to work on our own issues we erroneously embrace the belief that we are going to live forever. Choosing to stay numb to our pain we hold back joy from coming into our lives. Taking that extra muscle relaxer or the five or six Darvocet, Lortab, or Percocet a day to mask the pain numbs us even more.

Some folks do have to take such medicines on a regular basis to control their pain and remain functional, while others take the medicines because it's the easy thing to do, or because it is all that they know to do. During office visits, I hear, "I can't do anything. I have too much pain." My sense is that many of us are using our pain as an excuse to stay where we are and not venture into the unknown. We exercise our pain as an instrument to withhold our gifts to the rest of the world. By denying our power we close ourselves off to the greater good we have to offer. It is time to recognize that we all have a personal responsibility to live with greater awareness even though it may mean waking up to our own pain.

To these individuals I offer the following: If you were strong enough to get to the office, short of being on a stretcher, you have more power than you know to help yourself, but you have to take the time. If you can raise your foot an inch off the ground you can exert a minimal amount of extra effort and raise that foot two inches off the ground today. In a week with daily practice you will be able to raise the leg and foot four or five inches off the floor. From there you can proceed to work on other muscle groups using your will and mind to develop greater internal power. Our old beliefs keep us feeling helpless and stuck. Investing more energy into these beliefs to maintain them will only make us weaker with time.

When we attend to and focus on a particular muscle group, simple exercises can bring strength to that part of our body. Many of my patients complain that they are weak in the legs and have a hard time getting out of a chair. I sit beside them, take off my shoes and show them two easy exercises they can do four or five times a day for five minutes at a time. These exercises will help anyone develop strength in the quadriceps muscles. The key is to decide to take the time and do the work with intention.

At first when showing the range of motion they need to achieve, they passively swing their leg or foot with minimal effort. I have them engage the muscles of the lower legs by first having them spread out the toes. It is amazing to see how many people who cannot spread the fifth toe. I explain that the muscles in the lateral compartment of the lower leg have gone so long without being asked to perform that now they are asleep and don't want to be bothered. When a patient sees this for the first time it is like a light bulb goes off in their mind and they can see again. They are then instructed to imagine that they can spread the toe and intentionally ask the brain to tell the muscle to move. With time it will.

Once they understand how to activate the lower leg muscles, even though they may not be able to perform this simple act today, they are then asked to extend the leg straight removing the bend in the knee. Most of my patients cannot perform this movement because of weakness in the quads or anterior thigh muscles. In doing this movement they are instructed to keep the back straight and not lean backward. Once they get their leg to maximum extension, I have them hold it there as they continue to breathe slowly. With gentle encouragement they are instructed to contract the muscles of the anterior thigh. With the toes still engaged they are then directed to slowly bring the leg back down then start over with the other foot and leg.

The above exercise is so simple, but will only work if you take the time to do it. In the beginning you will actually sweat if you are doing it with the proper intention. Five minutes, two or three times a day, will strengthen the quads and make it easier to get out of a chair, easier to walk, and easier to stay balanced. In the right frame of mind, using this short time for self-exploration can be the beginning of a life-long journey that will open the widows of awareness.

By questioning our concept of time we can learn to expand time just as we can consciously ask our sleeping muscles to wake up and perform. We choose for ourselves what ideas, thoughts, feelings, and activities will fill our time. A little over a year ago I met an elderly, though otherwise previously healthy, man who developed a melanoma (a potentially lethal skin cancer) on the side of his neck. The tumor was removed, but because it had an unacceptable depth of penetration into the skin, he was offered a year of immune therapy using interferon. This required multiple trips to the office, but he did very well with the injections, experiencing minimal to nonexistent fatigue, no diarrhea, and no dangerous drop in his blood counts.

Two to three months after he completed the therapy he came in for follow-up and pointed out a new nodule on the neck, a large mass on his lower back, and a lesion on the roof of his mouth. The melanoma had returned at an aggressive pace. We had a discussion concerning potential therapeutic options, none of which were very hopeful. Many young individuals with metastatic melanoma will opt for chemotherapy in the hope that they will be one of the few who respond long-term, but this patient chose to withhold any further treatment and live out his days hoping for the best quality of life possible. He knew his time was limited and he was going to make the most of it visiting with friends, going out to lunch, and resting at home. Since he had not been previously ill, he felt especially blessed and peacefully accepted his fate.

He came in periodically to discuss pain management issues and on his last office visit, in which he carried himself in and out of on his own power, he said his final good-byes to the staff. He knew the end was near but he remained cheerful and determined to enjoy every minute that he had left. He felt no need to return knowing that hospice would be available to help him at home. His appreciation of the time and health he had been given up to his diagnosis made all the difference for him and his loved ones.

When we are experiencing difficult situations time seems to almost stand still. Mondays feel like the longest day of the week after returning to work following a weekend off. Our attitudes about work and challenges color the perception of time, but becoming aware of this we can consciously transform a second into a lifetime. Knowing that this moment is the only time we really have, we can resonate with life by staying in the moment.

The breath, as well as our attitude, are the instruments we use to remain in the moment. When we are worried or anxious over some future event we cannot appreciate the time that we have now. With our thoughts racing, our rapid breathing tries to keep up the pace. If we tell our minds to slow down, without the aid of the breath it won't happen. What makes us anxious in the first place is the fear of the unknown. When we perceive that we have no control over future events, we tense up, worry, and some develop panic attacks. When pain is a persistent visitor, anxiety, feelings of doom, and cat-astrophizing take hold and prevent us from staying in the present. Our only hope seems to be the wish that we will be pain free at some future time.

The following meditation will help to bring your consciousness into the moment and will assist in expanding the perception of time. Go to your quiet place. On the floor, carpeted is best, place a rolled blanket or quilt where lying on your back, you can drape your knees over it. Let the legs splay open with the feet falling to the sides in a relaxed manner. To support the head, place a cylindrical pillow, neck bolster, or a rolled towel under your neck. Place your arms, with the palms facing up, at a forty-five degree angle from your body. Allow your body to sink into the floor. Trust that the floor will support you and release all conscious muscular tension. Let the breath flow easily and observe it until it begins to undulate smoothly. Feel the rise and fall of the belly with the movement of the breath.

Once the mind begins to unwind, pinpoint the place on your body where you are experiencing the greatest pain. This may be a nagging tightness, a pulling or tugging sensation, a burning, searing feeling, or an acute sharp unbearable tearing stimulus. If it is the latter, back off and move to an area that is less intense. Having located your pain area, observe the pain and feel it the best you can without trying to change it in any way. This may be diffi-cult because our instinct is to immediately try and do something to alleviate or avoid such painful sensations. Resist the urge to move away from your pain. Be courageous and look at the pain. Feel its heat. Be bold and breathe into this pain even though this action may first increase its intensity. By employing the breath, you are becoming more aware of your pain, but with the direction of the breath, you are also intentionally increasing blood flow and needed oxygen to that previously deprived area.

With this heightened awareness, feel if you can pinpoint which muscle group or groups are squeezing down and contributing to and maintaining the pain. Those of us who suffer from TMJ will find incredible pressure coming from the massater, or chewing muscles. With the belly rising and falling, continue to direct the breath to the epicenter of your pain. As extraneous thoughts arise simply observe them and allow them to pass without being taken in by them. As fear or dread of the pain arises try to watch these impulses and observe the relationship between the body and the mind. With time you will be able to do all of this with greater ease and less apprehension, but you have to be willing to trust the process.

If you find things are becoming too intense, stop and take a break, and try again tomorrow. If you can stay with these sensations move on to the next step. Ask yourself, what is the purpose of this pain? What are you trying to protect yourself from? What belief lies behind this pain? See if you can determine if you are holding yourself responsible for something that you have no control over. Answers may not appear right away and it may take days, weeks, months, or years to get to the truth, but you will walk away with greater awareness of who you are and what forces are working on and through you.

When you get to the place where you feel that you have done enough for a day, once again focus your mind on the movement of the belly as the breath comes and goes. On the exhalation tell yourself that you are releasing all concerns out into the universe. On the inhalation tell yourself that you are receiving that which you need for total healing.

There is no need to rush in any of the work we are discussing. Many of us have jobs that create continuous external pressures that we have to contend with. Taking the time to practice the exercises in this book, in the quite of your own mind and away from the usual activities of the day, allows us to bring the insights gained through the practices into the world of our days. As we incorporate the teaching from within we find that events that do not fit into our new consciousness will fall away and they will no longer have the power to keep us stuck on the same wheel of existence.

Any sense of urgency should be dealt with in the quite of our meditation time. As you become more familiar with your internal landscape you will find that events will unfold as you have always wanted them to once you allow yourself to release the ideas of who you think you are. Coming into the present moment brings you to a new starting point, a point that has the potential to renew with each rising thought. The key is to not get hung up in beliefs that you have chosen to be your reality. Our reality is that we continually create our own reality every single minute of every day. It is when we lose sight of this fact that we become stuck and find ourselves lost in the time of the past.

The pain that we experience may have been with us for years but once we change our perspective about our pain and realize the contribution that we make that allows the continuation and the propagation of the pain then we can make readjustments. In a moment we open ourselves and see that maybe we don't have to hold on to this pain any longer. It has served us in the past, for whatever reason, but now seeing that it's usefulness is no longer helping, it is time to let it go. Do not be afraid of the emptiness that you think will follow. It is in this emptiness that new life will come. New ideas will fill your mind and new possibilities will arise. It is up to us to chose which way we will go.

In choosing to work against the clock we unknowingly push and contort our minds and bodies into places that are not healthy for us over time. Forcing ourselves to go to jobs that we dislike, or that drain the life energy out of us, sets the groundwork for a mindset that begins to feel at home in a pain-racked body. Only knowing pressure and finding motivation in "have to" situations allows internal anger to build. Lacking an outlet this anger is then turned inward and depression follows. Denial of the self leads only to greater pain. It separates us from others, keeps us awake at night, makes us irritable, and leaves no room for joy in our lives.

What a difficult lesson to learn. I my line of work I am always seeing people who have worked hard all their lives and then wake up one day to find that they have cancer. In the 15 years that I have been practicing oncology I have seen just one individual who I felt was totally satisfied with his life. He was in his early fifties and had metastatic colon cancer. His liver was full of cancer, as was his abdominal cavity. He was treated on a clinical trial but his cancer was discovered too late for any treatment to do any good. He came in for follow-up and enjoyed his time even to the end. His attitude remained one of appreciation. His words were genuine and he had no doubts about how he felt. His family did not understand his willingness to accept things just the way they were, but he knew himself and was happy for the experiences he had known and the life he was still living. The memorable thing about him was that he had no reservations of leaving this world. He innately trusted that what was on the other side for him was going to be just as good as what he was leaving. For him there was no time. No today, no tomorrow, no when this happens or when that happens. There was only now and he was in it. Over the few short weeks that I knew him, his family became more comfortable with where he was and a great deal of their anxiety lessened. To me, this man was a living meditation. He never really practiced a formal school of meditation but he was gifted in the fact that he was able to live his days one at a time no matter how things appeared from the outside.

When I learn of someone dying early, especially someone younger than I am, it makes me wonder just how much time I have left. This past weekend a young man we knew died prematurely. He left his home Friday evening to go bowling, mentioning to his wife that he would return around midnight. He was in good health, worked full time, was not overweight, and did not smoke or drink alcohol in excess. He had a loving wife of thirteen years and played joyfully with his two children, a six-year-old daughter and a three-year-old son. His picture was recently in the local newspaper, proudly displaying the eight-point buck he bagged, his first of the season. He looked and acted the picture of health. That night bowling, after he rolled a bad ball, he walked to the bench, sat down, and put his head in his hands. A few minutes later he was seizing. After forty minutes of attempted resuscitation he was pronounced dead.

His wife's greatest source of pain is the fact that she will never again be able to touch him. I feel for his wife who has days of uncertainty ahead. I feel compassion for his two children. His death makes me wonder what it might be like for my two boys if Treva or I were to die suddenly.   John

Trey, our eldest, would have a more difficult time and Joel would just wonder where his Daddy went. For a couple of weeks he would probably ask when is his Daddy coming home?

Our influence as parents is so great. The self-confidence and sense of trust that our children develop is directly related to how we view and interact with our children. Growing up with a harsh dad or a dad who isn't there emotionally may or may not be better than growing up without a dad. For these individuals, in order to heal, it will take a great deal of time and directed effort to overcome such a loss. They will have to learn to be their own fathers and once they become fathers they will have to possess the willingness and strength to learn the art of being there as a dad.

For someone who loses a parent early on, I can only imagine that they grow up wondering what it might have been like if they had never lost their parent. It is like someone took their lives and blew a huge hole into half of what they knew. All hopes of the future zapped and no one ever able to replace the loss. Those not directly affected by the loss wonder what the wife and kids are going through, but as the days pass our thoughts go less and less toward what the family has to face and more and more back to our own problems.

Another friend of mine lost his dad when he was only eleven years old. He spent fifteen years working through the pain of his loss. For him time was the healer, but also his pain had helped him to decide to become a healer. Working in chiropractic medicine he attends to those in pain as a result of accidents, arthritis, aging, and just not knowing any better on how to care for the body as we move along our journey. We all have places in our physical bodies where we allow the tensions of the day to build. These places will heal only when we begin to recognize that we are the one's who fail to discharge these energies and we are the one's who maintain these same energies through choosing to hold on to old beliefs about ourselves, our world, and our ideas about time.

Here is our wake up call. Let's not forget that no one is going to be here forever. It is a time to ask ourselves some pointed questions. Are we living the life that we have always wanted for ourselves, doing what we love and what feeds us? If not, then it is time to do some serious thinking, look at our priorities and make some changes. Priorities do change and it is good to question if we are living the life we thought we should be living or if we are just putting up with things in the hope that things will get better later. The death of the young man makes me think that for some of us there may not be much time left. We just never know when our time is up. When we leave the house to go to work, or when we drive to the grocery store there is no guarantee that we will ever come home. We take our lives for granted.

In order to develop a renewed appreciation for what we have been given it is essential to remain centered in the moment. Richard Carlson and Joseph Bailey tell us in *Slowing Down to the Speed of Life: How to Create a More Peaceful, Simpler Life From the Inside Out*:

> "When we are able to remain centered in the moment, in our relationships, we experience: intimacy, joy, spontaneity, play, deep listening, effective communication, respect, compassion, empathy, kindness, openness, and gratitude."[1]

Our decision and commitment to listen to our inner voices from the place of quiet meditation becomes the stepping stone to the path of greater inner peace and being. The possibility of overcoming any and all obstacles to optimum health exists for all of us and this truth will be made real in your life once you open your mind to hearing it. Your pain, frustration, and anger are messengers that are telling you that you are out of balance and it is time to take a stand and listen to their message. We have a choice to continue on with our current level of pain and discomfort and keep doing what we have been to cope, or we can chose to take responsibility for what we experience and take the steps to begin meditation and yoga and in doing so, grow in awareness and balance.

In Stephen Levine's book, *One Year to Live*, his research led him to discover that most people said they would slow down at work if they knew they had only one year left to live. Many said they would quit their jobs feeling they would devote the little time left to pursuits they had always wanted to follow. When people were told they had one year to live, many discovered a new spaciousness they had not previously known. Social status dropped as one of their priorities. Relationships that were going nowhere were allowed to die and there was a renewed desire to really live and do what moved them.

I remember going to school as a young boy and then later into high school and college. Medical school, internship, residency and finally the last three years of training in Hematology/Oncology followed. All through those years the goal was to be someone, someone who people wanted to talk with and listen to. Living for the future, I lived for the day when I could say that I had made it, when I called the shots, and did what I wanted.

It was a sacrifice but I got what I wanted. It has been difficult to turn off the attitude of living for the future. Living and working all of those years in this deeply ingrained attitude cannot be turned off with the snap of the fingers. In my meditation and yoga I find myself working to undo what I have done to myself but I find that my muscles, my fascia, and my entire makeup are frozen in past beliefs and this results in physical pain. It takes conscious effort to try and move my fascia and musculature back to where nature meant them to be instead of in the forced position I find myself in all of the time. Consciously teasing the muscles to loosen, like someone would tease a knotted string is the only way to get them to release past conditioning. During the yoga asanas and associated breathing, the muscles reluctantly give up their old memories and move into a place of newness yet uncertainty. It's pick and pull, pick and pull. Pull one part of the string to try and tease another part to loosen up. As I do that another part of me tightens up in response. It is the discipline gained from meditation that allows my mind to remain calm and concentrated on the task at hand as I move slowly toward greater balance with each moment of practice.

Breathing into a muscle and feeling the heat in that muscle as some of the sensation begins to return helps bring some life back to it. Watching my right arm and hand tremble as I tell them to relax and breathing into the muscles of my neck and shoulder, I wonder if I am going to be an old man someday, unable to drink his morning cup of coffee because of uncontrollable trembling. My motivations have changed. I do not want to be a shaky old man. I do not want to live in constant pain. Who would want such a life? Many people live in such a state but the price they pay is a life without feeling.

We all try to cover up our deficiencies. If we truly knew that we had only one year to live we would not expend our energies in such vain pursuits. Growing up we always ponder over what we want to be when we grow up. Instead as we grow in wisdom, a healthier attitude to assume is to just enjoy life and time with our families and friends. Maybe I'm shifting gears because I'm over fifty. Maybe my meditation and spiritual pursuits are beginning to pay off. We can all undergo a paradigm shift and see our fear yet not let it paralyze us. Centering in meditation allows us to sit with whatever comes up. Instead of fleeing from our fears we can say, "Oh, I wonder what that's all about?" This will bring us back to center and back into the now, away from the fantasies of the past. We can see that it's not going to be that bad. Maybe we can all get the to point someday when we can say that death is not going to be so bad. It will take work and conscious effort but in the end it should make our own deaths easier to deal with.

Last night we, as a family, attended the young man's funeral. The local funeral home has taken a step into the high tech realm. They take home photographs and put them onto a DVD and run the disc on a TV screen for all to see. We stood watching photos flash by, showing a thrilled boy taking his first independent ride on his two-wheeler while his Dad, just as excited, looks on. Dad's arms are spread out wide at his sides, while he runs along with his son, both jubilant. This one photo bought a tear to my eye. I know what it is like to watch my son take his first ride alone. It is a milestone, a step of independence. It is an affirmation that everything to date has been done right. All of the effort, all of the patience has paid off. Our boys have become boys. No longer toddlers they are moving into the next phase.

To know the young boy will not have his Dad around when he learns to drive and takes the car out on his own for the first time hurts. To know that his Dad will not be there for his preschool graduation or his grade school and high school graduation is painful. To know that six year old little girl will not be given away by her Dad when she gets married brings an emptiness to my heart. Even tougher to deal with is the knowledge that the young boy will probably not remember much of his encounters with his Dad.

Life is short for those of us who live an expected life expectancy. It is even shorter for those of us who die prematurely. No one knows what the main game plan is. We can only hope that whatever amount of time that we have here is useful in some way to others.

Walking into the viewing room I had an image of my own funeral. Looking at the beautiful flower arrangements with the bright red carnations, the white roses, and inhaling their fragrances I wondered what people might say about me after my death. If we could stand in on a conversation between our spouse and family, or between our spouse and friends, or children and co-workers and neighbors, what would we hear? Will we be missed? Will there be relief for the survivors, as I had a sense of relief after my mother's death because she had been ill for so many years? Will others say we were whiners, or complainers? Would we hear them talk about how hard we worked or how hard we tried to do the right thing? Will they say that we were a good husband or wife and a good mother or father? Will the general theme revolve around how well we had lived or how hard we had struggled?

If we seriously consider some of these questions now and look ahead to a time after our own passing we can affect change in our lives. When these conversations do come to pass, and they will for everyone, then the talk will be positive. People will miss us and be glad that we walked this earth and crossed their paths.

On reflecting about death I think about the life of my mother. She died at a relatively young age. With all of her deficiencies she did give me life and she raised me to the best of her ability. When she first went into the hospital my father had adequate insurance. We would visit her in the evenings and on weekends. We would visit for 30-45 minutes. The hospital had a large recreation room with full window walls. Families could sit with their hospitalized relatives and Dads would talk with Dads and compare notes, telling each other's reasons for the hospitalization. They talked about events leading up to the hospitalization and what they were hoping for in the future.

After the insurance money ran out, my mother was placed in the state hospital. Young children were not allowed to visit. We would drive the fifty minutes to Middletown with our father and wait in the car while he visited for half an hour. We were kids and didn't really know much of what was going on. Still we made the best of our time together and waited, joking around in the parking lot. The "thirty-five cent" man would come along ask-

41

ing us for money for cigarettes. He was one of the inpatients who roamed the grounds. Of course we had no money to give him, but we got a lot of mileage out of his line for years after.

My mother eventually died in a nursing home while in her mid-50's. She never came home to live again, but on good days, when she felt better, my father would pick her up after work and she would have dinner with us. Now twenty years after her death, I am beginning to try to piece her life, or what I knew of it, together.

There is no reason for us to act like kids when it comes to death. If we think by ignoring the issue that it is going to go away, then we are in for a surprise. We have to prepare for death and look at it as a natural event in our lives. Because we spend time thinking about it does not mean that we have a wish to die. It just means that we want to be realistic and be ready for it. The more we can prepare, the more our families can accept it when it comes for us. I have seen such preparation lessen the suffering. Thinking about what life will be like after a spouse is gone is not morbid. The occasional glimpse into the future may give us a sense of peace, or a sense of completion.

Such walks with death might help us look out our windows at sunset and really see the baby blue in the sky. Maybe we'll see the soft pink clouds acting as contrast for the purple-gray clouds lying closer to the horizon. These glimpses of death may allow us to hear our own breath. We may not only hear the flow of life giving oxygen flowing through our airways, but we may feel the light coolness of the in-breath as it rushes into the back of our throat and raises our chest to meet the heavens.

As the day dies at sunset, we come to a place where we experience the quietest time of the day. We can hope that at the time of our death it will also be quite and peaceful. Looking at death in this way gives us the opportunity, the desire, the reason, to live now. To live in full appreciation of what we now experience. With the knowledge that all of this will pass, we are more likely to take fewer things for granted and want to be a part of what is here now. Fear does not have to be invited. This gift of life is just that.

With the recent death so close, and our boys knowing the two children of the deceased, Treva wanted to help John Trey and Joel understand more about death. She wanted to do it in a soft and non-threatening way. She decided to borrow a video from friends of ours: *The Lion King*. As you recall Mufasa, the proud lion king had a cub named Simba. Simba's uncle, jealous of Mufasa, planned and executed the death of Mufasa but in the process made young Simba feel that he was responsible for his father's death. Simba was told by his uncle to run away and never come back. He eventually returned with the help of Rafiki, a wise baboon, to reclaim his place in the circle of life. He grew up learning that his father would live his life then die, he would live his life and die, and his son would do the same. The boys were able to see the cycle of son to father repeated. It is never too young to begin living with the knowledge of our own mortality. This knowledge gives us reason to live everyday as if it were our last.

Section Two

FINDING YOUR FIRE

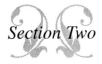

Section Two

FINDING YOUR FIRE

Introduction

*I*t takes an incredible amount of energy to hide who we really are. Imagine all that could be accomplished if the dispersed energy that we expend could be focused and directed toward developing a sense of wholeness and completeness. As we move through the next three chapters we will explore the ways that our internal energies can be brought into greater balance through the study of the ancient Chakra system.

The Chakras are energy centers that we all possess. They have specific anatomical locations as well as specific physical, psychological, and emotional connotations. Depending on which energy centers are out of balance there will be deficiencies in such areas as feeling a part of the community, inferiority issues, difficulties with making our needs known, and an inability to see ahead, plan, and thus manifest what we are here to do. The following pages will foster a working knowledge of this ancient system that we can use daily to maintain our sense of balance in all of our undertakings.

As we steadily work through the issues that bother us the most, nuggets of insight will begin to move into our field of thought. There will come a time when a major shift in attitude will occur and problems will be viewed as a means to become more present. This awareness makes itself known as we begin to acknowledge that our pain is truly trying to tell us something and that it is not a punishment for some past misdeed we may have done out of ignorance. As we tell ourselves that it is safe to listen, that there is no need to run from the pain, we realize that it is possible to make space for pain, to go on with the pain, and even at times to notice that the pain is actually absent. The following chapters will lead us on the quest for the gold that survives the trials by fire.

In the meditative exercises that follow we will experience long lost insights that will assist in differentiating real past injuries from exaggerated scenarios that have been carried as excess baggage for years. It is in this non-reactive state that healing takes place.

As the practice of meditation matures we will learn to sit with the things that scare us and do so with courage. Even though the flames of the fire are barely visible and all that we can see are the dying embers as a result of longstanding depression, with breath work or pranayama practice the flames will again emerge and be put to constructive use. We will find that the fire becomes the source of energy to live our passions.

The Seven Major Spinal Chakras

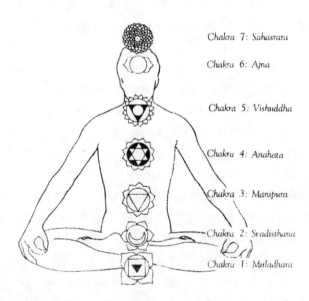

Chakra 7: Sahasrara

Chakra 6: Ajna

Chakra 5: Vishuddha

Chakra 4: Anahata

Chakra 3: Manipura

Chakra 2: Svadisthana

Chakra 1: Muladhara

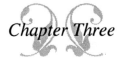

Chapter Three

Discovering New Sources of Energy

*A*mericans are suffering. Life is full of suffering all over the world. We can consider ourselves fortunate that we do not live in Iraq or the Sudan, but we add to our own misery by not recognizing the power that we have to affect positive change in our lives and in the lives of those we love.

It is estimated that 500,000 Americans suffer from chronic fatigue. This is a syndrome manifested by severe unexplained chronic fatigue for greater than six months. Other associated symptoms may include impairment of short-term memory or concentration, muscle pain, joint pain, headache, and lack of restful sleep.[1] The persistent lack of energy can lead to burnout and depression. With the never-ending fatigue, all hope for living a satisfying life is lost. As the symptom complex continues your inner circle contracts, leaving you wallowing in loneliness, pain, and defeat.

Even greater numbers of Americans are dealing with the ravages of depression. Practicing acceptance in these conditions only goes so far. It doesn't lead to greater joy or allow for increasing rays of hope for healing. Feeling left out and ignored, the only appropriate recourse seems to be to live with it and take your beating. Antidepressants can help to a degree, but they also have a way of numbing the mind, thus removing you from directly experiencing the joys in life.

Many times our attitudes and beliefs are repressive and inhibit us from thinking our way out of our webs. To remain with old beliefs is to resign yourself to further pain and torment. On the other hand, to take a chance and do something different, or to choose to look at things from another perspective, will lead you back to the on-ramp of life. It's time to leave the untended rest stop and venture out to where you have never allowed yourself to go. It will be scary at times, but so what. If it gets your heart beating faster and makes your breathing deeper, then more power to you. You have more energy than you think and there is more energy floating around all of us to go around. By learning a few simple techniques and by changing your perspective on a few ideas, this energy will flow to you freely and upon demand.

From great minds like Einstein to Carl Sagan, it is believed that we all come from the same carbon atoms. Five billion years ago, at the time of the big bang, all the currently existing atoms were created. As the laws of physics tell us, the amount of energy in the universe is constant and energy is neither created nor destroyed. It is transformed from one state to another. We each share the same atoms that were part of the world from the beginning, thus even though we may look different on the outside; we are all the same on the inside.

Individuals who believe in such theory are referred to as atomists, believing that all things are made of atoms. In chemistry we study the periodic table and the relationship that each element has to each other. We also know about orbits and the spin that an electron undergoes in relation to its nucleus. We understand that there are different energy levels that an electron jumps to depending on the amount of energy in the system. We are charged just as the individual atoms that form our most basic building blocks are. That we can affect and influence these energy systems buried within are ideas not entertained by the masses. I intend to bring some light onto the power that we each possess over our own energy systems. It may be a power that until now many of us have been afraid to approach. The reason for understanding and working with these energy systems is to help us create and integrate wholeness within ourselves, to find inner balance, and to move in a direction of decreasing our own pain

In choosing not to recognize our own energies we shut ourselves down. We unknowingly make our lives more difficult than they have to be and create more problems than solutions. With the life force shut out, we wonder why we are not enjoying life and not getting what we want.

The ancients used a system based on energy centers within the body. Dating as far back as Egyptian times man has been studying and working with the Chakra System. There are seven main chakras within the body as well as multiple sub-chakras. The word Chakra is a Sanskrit word meaning wheel. These "wheels" are located near sympathetic ganglia within our central nervous systems. The chakras function like the lens of a camera in that they can open and close. When the chakras are in balance one's life is in balance. If a chakra or multiple chakras are closed or blocked, then an individual will experience lack in a corresponding area of their life. Chakras interact with each other within the body and interact with the chakras of other individuals.[2]

Each of the chakras corresponds with particular body organs as well as with emotional and psychological patterns. Disease will appear in the energy system first before manifesting in the physical body. One can practice preventative medicine by clearing the system with grounding techniques or daily meditation. This mind-body medicine focuses on the needs and rhythm of the body as well as the pulse of the soul. It is unfortunate that each of us living and working in modern day life is too busy to pay attention to our mind-body connection. This is to our detriment, but by practicing yoga or sitting in meditation, even in small increments, we can educate ourselves and tune into our landscape.

One of the first ways to begin to notice your own energy field is by palpation. Go to a quite place, and start by practicing three-part breathing. After quieting the mind, slowly bring your palms into proximity. As they come within ten to twelve inches of each other you will feel a gentle repulsion, like some force is trying to keep the hands apart. That force is your energy field. You will notice it getting larger the more you attend to it.

Being able to sense your own energy field is similar to having the feeling that someone is watching or staring at you. We are going along minding our own business when a strange feeling overcomes us. We look around and someone is watching us or trying to get our attention. We did not use any of our five usual senses to pick this up, but instead we were feeling higher energy vibrations.

As stated above, our chakras interact with the chakras of others. The interaction takes place through string or ribbon-like lines of energy called cords. They penetrate another's chakra to connect individuals on an energetic level. There are good cords, necessary for healthy interaction, as well as bad cords, which lead to dependency, and dysfunctional interaction. Both types are a person's request for attention. A cord between a mother and her infant child at the first chakra allows for caring and survival of the child as the first chakra (root chakra) has to do with our being and our getting along on this planet. It is our connection to mother earth and our connection with our tribe as a member of the human race. It also signifies our place in our community and at a closer level our interaction with our own families. The first chakra is located in the area of the lower spine. In men the general location is at the base of the spine whereas in women it is located in the area between the ovaries.

The second chakra is found around the navel area. This is where we perceive other people's emotions and where we sense what other people are feeling. Our capacity to empathize is located in this chakra. The quality of day-to-day interaction is determined by the health of the second chakra. Balanced in the second chakra we find ourselves fortunate in having balanced relationships with others. Exhaustive states resulting from dependency issues or care-taking are minimized. A healthy interaction between the second and fifth chakra plays a role in the creative process allowing us to seemingly make something from nothing.

The third chakra is our center of self-esteem. It is where our sense of whom we are to ourselves resides. When in balance we are able to go through life and face daily challenges with confidence. When blocked it seems that there is nothing we can do right, nothing comes easy and we go through life afraid of everything. As Deedre Diemer explains in her book *The ABC's of Chakra Therapy*, a cord in the third chakra means, "I want some of your energy, my own is not enough."[3] In dealing with cancer patients or for that matter anyone who has a terminal diagnosis, their energy stores are depleted and they are searching for others to be a source of strength. They are intuitively aware that in order to have quality of life they need energy. Today many clinical studies that evaluate the effectiveness of new therapies have a component that assesses the quality of life a patient experiences during treatment. A health care provider or a family member caring for those with terminal disease or a disease that requires intensive therapy needs to be aware that their energy flow is directed away from center. By being aware that the patient pulls energy, it is possible to take the necessary steps to recharge. The recharging process can be as easy as taking a few moments to ground with the earth. This can be done even when tending to the patient.

A very simple technique to use for immediate grounding involves using our imagination to picture a wire or cable running from the root chakra and connecting to the center of the earth. The cable can be connected to the core of the earth in any fashion. I like to imagine the cable grabbing on to the center of the earth, which is mostly iron, through a giant electromagnet. With this vision in mind we are able to draw energy from the earth and we are not letting this precious energy dispel itself through the top of our heads. The conscious recognition of our presence in the here and now enables us to vibrate in the moment and be a part of the ubiquitous ever moving energy.

Using the breath to release negative energy is a technique that can also be done at any time. When I visit my local acupuncturist the first thing that he does upon entering the treatment room is to take a deliberate, slow exhalation through pursed lips. It is his way of clearing the field for his energy work to take hold and a way that he can protect himself from the discordant energy he encounters in his patients. It takes some time to master the process but once learned it can be used at any time or in any situation in which one is being stressed.

The breath is a powerful tool that can be used to move energy through the body. It can open up tight muscles and can be used to mobilize fascia. When awareness is brought to a tight muscle, consciously breathing into that muscle and feeling the postural change created by the movement of the oxygen, the muscle cannot help but loosen and relax, that is if you are willing to let this happen. On the out-breath the spine and neck can be made more erect and this also facilitates the movement of oxygen. The result is a more relaxed state of being and a feeling of oneness with the environment.

The fourth chakra is the heart chakra. Located in the region of our physical heart it has to do with compassion and nurturance. An open fourth chakra gives us a sense of oneness with life and the ability to receive and give unconditional love. One closes the fourth chakra when there has been a number of real or perceived hurts though out life that have not been dealt with. Closing down the heart chakra is felt as a tightness or holding on in the left chest area. There can be asymmetry in the pectoralis major and minor muscles, which are located in the upper chest. The posture of an individual with a closed fourth chakra will have them bending forward in an effort to further protect their heart from greater pain. There are many wonderful people in the world who are capable and willing to give their love to others but in order to receive this love one needs to keep the heart chakra open. In protecting the heart from further hurt, closing down this chakra effectively prevents any good from coming in.

The fifth chakra, or the throat chakra, has to do with communication. It is literally our inner voice. When functioning properly it allows us to take care of our personal needs. This chakra also plays a role in the creative process in that when listening to the inner voice we allow ourselves to connect with the wisdom that is always there. As the eyes are the windows to the world, the throat is the window to universal wisdom. The throat, being between the head and the heart, will either allow the two areas to stay connected or will help prevent communication between the two. When there is great sadness and great hurt within the heart area, the head or the "I" within does not want to know that pain. In this respect the neck tenses and squeezes down thus closing the throat chakra.

The beauty of the system is that we are in control of all of this. The problem is that in our efforts to protect ourselves from the pain we choose to forget this fact and allow the pain to continue. This is why self-awareness and awareness of the body-mind connection is so important to health and well being. Muscle has memory and fascia has memory. It will do us well to remember this. Everyone thinks that all of our higher functions take place in the brain. Why, in a system as complex as the human body, would anyone think that one area and one area alone would control everything? When we think this then disease occurs. We are an integrated system where all parts contribute to the healthy functioning of the whole.

Moving on to the sixth chakra, we find that it is located between the eyebrows. Otherwise known as the third eye, the sixth chakra has to do with clear seeing, intuition, personal vision, and wisdom. Healthy functioning of the third eye allows us to have clarity in our life's vision. We know what we are doing and why we are doing it. We can see where we are going and we are going there because we want to and not because someone else wants us to.

The seventh chakra is located at the top of the head. An open seventh chakra allows us to see our larger purpose. It is the chakra that permits free will, giving us faith in our being. It has to do with values, ethics, courage, and humanitarianism. In the health care profession we all act as humanitarians, caring for those in need, even on days when we feel that we need some care. We are in a position of putting the other person first all of the time. With the balance that is natural from healthy functioning chakras we are able to continue such pursuits knowing that balance is possible. We can assist others and at the same time we can meet our own needs. It happens by making the conscious decision that we are going to be bigger than what we see in front of us. There are techniques that we can learn which allow us to take care of others and at the same time take care of ourselves. The seventh chakra allows us to trust life and that process.

Last week I was seeing a patient for the first time. He had Hepatitis C infection of the liver and suffered from chronic depression. Looking past the depressed affect, he appeared to be a relatively healthy individual with good muscle mass. He did not demonstrate the telltale signs of malnutrition as he had an obvious lack of bitemportal muscle wasting. His major compliant was that he lacked energy. He denied having nightmares and slept a reasonable amount of time at night. He was taking Zoloft but no other anxietyolytics or sedatives.

As we talked his craving for more energy was palpable. The exam room that we were in has a small window at about shoulder height. As he lamented over his plight, my eye caught the movement of the branches and leaves of a birch tree. As he completed a sentence, I asked him to turn around and gaze upon the quivering movement of the leaves in the breeze. As we placed our attention on the dancing leaves, shivering rapidly like the feet of a *Riverdance* performer, I began to explain that we can feel the pulsation of energy all around us, if that is where we chose to put our focus. In a depressive state our attention is turned inward more often that outward. As our body slows, so does the mind, but when we reach out and feel and pay attention, we can experience the energy of the wind and make it ours, if even for a moment.

I have seen him in follow-up and he subjectively feels that he has more energy. I see that objectively, as he did not appear as downtrodden as he had on the first visit. Once we open up to this knowledge we are forever changed. Being able to consciously change our focus, especially when experiencing pain, be it pain from a slipped disc, fibromyalgia, arthritis, or bursitis, is a gift that we can accept whenever the need arises. Removing ourselves from our own internal aloneness, and opening ourselves to the energy all around us, we decrease our suffering.

Living in eastern North Carolina we are only two hours away from the Atlantic Ocean. In the summer months our town is deserted after 5 PM on Friday nights as everyone heads for the beach. Yesterday I saw an elderly lady in follow-up that had been treated for breast cancer over ten years ago. She was one of my first patients. She has done extremely well and has had no evidence of recurrence of the breast cancer. Her visit yesterday was related to the CAT scan guided biopsy of a mass in the left upper lobe of her lung. She had come in the previous week complaining of increasing weight loss and a productive cough. The cough was nothing new as she had been treated for bronchitis on multiple occasions in the past. Her weight loss and increasing fatigue is what led her daughter to bring her in for evaluation.

Her problem is that she loves her cigarettes more than she loves her life. During each office visit I have counseled her concerning giving up the smoking. Recently, I told her that she had the worst sounding lungs I have ever heard. She has such severe emphysema, that with auscultation, I could barely hear any air moving in and out of her lungs with each breath. It has finally come to pass that she now has lung cancer. Fortunately she has given up smoking and is doing fairly well.

In times of stress, or when she wants to get away from things for a while, she will go to Atlantic Beach and fish off the pier. To her there is nothing better than spending the day fishing and taking in the ocean air. She tells me this as she takes in a deep inhalation through flared nostrils. With the recent passing of hurricane Alex, she explains that she loves to be at the beach during a storm. She basks in the power of the wind, the wildness of the waves, and the ease with which it's energy allows her to breathe. It is as if the energy of the storm and the movement of the blustering winds take up her extra work of breathing and gives her a needed respite. She knows innately that the forces of nature will lessen her struggle and so wanted to be at the shore to have the winds blow through her and help her feel whole again this day.

The rhythmic splashing of the waves assists her in coming into balance with the frequency of the natural. All of her concerns being mind-made and worry oriented are cancelled out and flooded from consciousness by the pulse and purging propagation of the ocean. As we are mostly water, she vibrates in concert with her surroundings and thus lives in momentary harmony. Anyone who has ever crossed the bridges at Moorehead City or Emerald Isle to gain access to the island will tell you they experience a sigh of relief as they sense the water below them. The expanse of the water facilitates a deeper passage of the breath by encouraging a fuller, uninhibited inhalation, and a smoother, non-ratcheting exhalation that allows for complete emptying of the lungs. This release is performed without a desire for grasping and holding onto the breath.

It takes energy to grasp and continually hold on to the life force. We tire and fatigue by our unwillingness to let go of each breath. Fearful of losing it forever, we will struggle to keep what we have. When in close proximity to the incredible energy of the universe, as demonstrated by the ocean winds and waves, we remember that it is natural to let go. The next breath will come if it is meant to be, just as the next wave will come.

We are powerful beings but are constantly busy – rushing from here to there - often underestimating the change we can make in our lives. Change generates energy and when we resist change we have chosen to close ourselves to the energy that is available to us. Our preoccupied minds have the capacity to create just what we want and rid ourselves of what no longer serves us. The timetable may not always be to our liking, as creation takes patience and thought, but in honesty we receive what we think we deserve. We create and recreate our worlds every second of every day. Our dominant thoughts determine what we manifest. We can invest our energy into areas that will result in what we want or we can disperse and diffuse our energies and experience the heaviness of depression, fatigue, and chronic anxiety. In the meditative state we slow down enough, quite the chatter enough to see this fact clearly. In this place we can choose the middle way and allow the flow of energy to move through us and guide us and power us to meet our potential.

Everyone has the power and the know-how to make things happen. Even when told it can't be done, with patience and perseverance we can manifest what we desire.

Creativity is a process. In order to be as creative as possible we need to allow ourselves to trust our inner workings. We cannot be afraid of our own energy, but need to stay open to the inner voice, a voice that wants to tell us the best and easiest way for us to proceed. This voice knows all of the answers and will direct and lead us to a natural unfolding of events, thoughts and feelings. When we try to force events or conditions we get into trouble. We get tight and tense, locking and freezing the flow of internal energy. We feel pressured and have a need to get what we want when we want it now instead of allowing events to occur in their own time. Ease of effort comes when we allow ourselves to get into the flow of things. A book titled *Flow* by Mihaly Csikszentmihalyi describes flow states. In this state work seems effortless. Timelessness occurs and there is a sense of oneness with the activity. With the mind focused and concentrated, there is an absence of fatigue even when the work is intense. The creative process is facilitated by flow states. The mind, free from distraction, is allowed to express its hidden treasures.

We all have ideas, some better than others. Many times others reject our ideas, especially if they have more experience or seniority. We can look at our individual creativity instead and not worry about the group at first. When we are able to see improvement in our creative process the results of this process will naturally spill into all aspects of our lives. Others sensing our clarity will naturally want to support us.

The creative process can be learned just like one can learn to fly fish. Reading books on the topic, talking to others about the process and practicing all help to hone our creative skills. It is time to get creative in finding ways to overcome our pain.

In the book, *Creating*, by Robert Fritz, he points out that all of us have a "deep longing to create." The way to reach for the highest within us is by creation. We all have the tools needed to create. Fritz brings out the important point that creating is not problem solving though one can be creative in their approach at coming up with solutions to problems. When I was growing up in the 1960's and attending Bishop School and then Webster School, most of our time was spent doing programmed work as written out in the teacher's daily lesson plan. We spent hours doing math, reading, and spelling. The only "creative time" set aside was recess. It was playtime. We can look at our creative efforts as a sort of play. In yoga workshops that I have participated in with Rodney Yee, he has emphasized that we should try to take an attitude of playfulness as we practice. The last thing we want to do is to grit our teeth, furrow our foreheads, and clench our jaws while practicing yoga. It makes sense that to be able to enjoy any activity, be it playing baseball, working on a term paper or even getting a business contract together we do not need to insert our own ideas of how hard the task might be. That would only add to the work involved. Effort in anything is just that, putting out more than is necessary. Keeping a lighthearted, easy attitude about this may sound like we don't care about an issue. Such an attitude allows us to step back and see all aspects of a situation and not just our own limited take on an issue. It allows for the unimpeded flow of energy, a flow that feels good.

Toys are excellent tools that facilitate the creative process. My sons are forever playing with their Legos. Today there are giant Legos for children like Joel, my four year old. They are easier to manipulate than the smaller standard Legos that John Trey uses. Most of the Legos we buy come as kits to build airplanes or airports and basketball courts. There are Legos based on the Harry Potter stories. Not all of the Legos are predetermined to become something. It's the Legos that are scattered all over the room after a piece has been taken apart that are the greatest teaching tools. The guys and their friends create previously unimagined cars, boats, planes, and spacecraft by putting one piece together at a time. They focus their energies, look at what is available in front of them, and they build until their heart's content. Then they play with their new creations. For them it is play but what I see is the creative process being expressed and practiced.

In anything that is created we are constantly learning and adjusting our actions based on what is learned. In creating we cannot help but remain fluid and we facilitate the free movement of our energy. It is when we allow energy to stagnate that we permit our muscles to tighten, our brows to furrow, our breath to become shallow, and our pain to intensify. When we start looking at our life as the focus of our creative process we begin to change everything. It is as if we are able to get down to the molecular level of our beings and rearrange things the way we want them to be.

Last night on TV I caught the last half of "Nova." It was an episode titled, "The Elegant Universe." I learned about the string theory of the universe. Apparently the string theory has evolved over time into a membrane theory. Modern day physicists are attempting to explain a unified theory of the universe. The origin of mass is the basic question being explored. In the same light when we want to create we can ask, how do we manifest something from nothing? What energies are involved? A common belief among scientists is that we cannot create something from nothing. It is theorized that mass is created by a process called pelastration. Pelastration is a combination of penetration and elasticity. It occurs when a force penetrates an infinite stretchable flexible layer of space and carries part of the flexible layer beyond its own space. In simplest form creation is the movement of membrane tubes within tubes with these tubes having the capacity to create sub-tubes, coils and knots. Pelastration creates dimensions.

The analogy of the Uroboros, the serpent that swallows its own tail, best describes the process of pelastration. The snake swallows its tail once, then circles around again to swallow it's tail again. The leading edge breaks away from the snake proper able to cross and intersect at different points. The movement is all vibration or energy. When doing yoga, if we can experience the vibration of our bodies, the vibration of our muscles, the vibration of our being, then we are experiencing life and creation, and we are one with our own energy.

As Dirk Laureyssens, a leading researcher in membrane theory says, "Everything is connected to everything, it's only a question of amplitude, length, frequency, level, angle and position in the tube constellation. When one membrane tube embeds into another tube, with the movement of space, parts of that space can be doubled. An infinite elastic membrane surrounds the space. As these membranes roll onto themselves, unbreakable strings are created. These strings are the boundaries of newly created mass. It is believed that the subatomic particles we see in nature are different resonances of the vibrating superstrings. Resonances are movements that create internal friction. Different combinations of these vibrations create the basic particles of our universe. Our process of creating thoughts may somehow have the ability to cause these membranes to move in ways that they would not have moved without our intervening presence. This is our power to create. These membranes being interconnected tell us we are made of these same membranes and we are all one. The Uroboros not only symbolizes the renewal of the universe but also the integration of the shadow self and the power of the Kundalini which sits within the first chakra waiting to rise to the heavens.

In *A Complete Guide to Acupressure,* Iona Marsaa Teeguarden explains that the *Jing* in Chinese medicine is our "Essence, or the substance that underlies all organic life." *Jing* itself is supportive and nurtures us. *Jing* is different from *Qi* or pure energy, but *Jing* can be transformed into *Jing Qi,* or reserve energy. Some of our *Jing* is inherited and the remainder is obtained from the foods that we eat.[4]

Everyone is not born equal when it comes to *Jing.* Whenever there are other imbalances in the meridians, or energy pathways of the body, and their governing organs, *Jing* will be in deficiency. Teeguarden goes on to explain that the role of yoga is in "training, cultivating, and building the "Three Treasures," 1) *Jing,* or vital essence, which creates *Qi*; 2) *Qi,* or life force, which creates *Shen*; and 3) *Shen,* or spirit."

We come to the yoga asanas with the intention of experiencing the above, but we can't force ourselves to generate *Jing*, *Qi*, or *Shen*. This is where we have to take the instruction of the sage Patanjali who wrote over 2500 years ago in *The Yoga Sutras of Patanjali*, "while practicing *asana* release all effort and keep your mind focused on the infinite." Such focus gets our minds out of the way and allows the free movement of *Jing*, *Qi*, and *Shen*. The practice of three-part breathing that was reviewed earlier also energizes us because the *Qi* collects in the *Dantian* in the lower abdomen.

An acupuncturist will place needles in blocked points on a meridian as well as distal points along the same meridian. This complementary placement of the needles allows for the reinstitution of the flow of energy. At home we can use our fingers to apply pressure to these same points and do the same thing. An excellent book that shows the location of "trigger points," is *The Trigger Point Therapy Workbook: Your Self-Treatment Guide for Pain Relief.*[5]

What can you do if you happen to be one of the individuals who never had any significant amount of energy as noted in those who are born deficient in *Jing*? If you are reading this, chances are you want more energy and you know what it's like to live with fatigue. You, more than likely, have had to push to get anything done in your life. You may feel that you have no energy for the enjoyment of even the littlest things and may feel cheated and passed over.

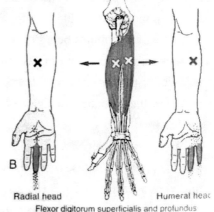

Radial head   Humeral head
Flexor digitorum superficialis and profundus

Carpal tunnel trigger points

In order to begin to experience increasing energy you will need to feel what you have been afraid to look at up to now. The lack of energy is fertile ground for envy, jealousy, anger, and their resultant pain associations. In your quiet place, look back to a time when you were engrossed in an activity that consumed your energies. What were you doing at the time and what were your underlying feelings? Wait for an image, or a feeling to arise. When it does try not to shut down, but breathe easily and experience the feeling even if you have to "see" it as an outside observer. If the feeling that arises is sadness, then feel the sadness. If it is extreme, stay with it until you can generate a sense of compassion for yourself. If, when the image comes up, you feel that you will never get over it, or that it is too complex to resolve in the moment, then radiate compassion for yourself and anyone else who you know has had a rough time. Until you are able to feel your hidden feelings, you will keep your energy tied up in repressing your pain. Facing the fear and allowing yourself to feel will get your life force moving again so that you can feel like you belong again.

If you were a caring adult watching the above unfold, what would you say to the one who is suffering? It is healthy to feel what you are feeling, even if the feelings are construed as being negative. Do not beat yourself up. You did what you had to do in the past to survive. Your defenses served you well, but now that they are causing you pain and draining you constantly, it is time to acknowledge them and let them go. Trust yourself to know what to do.

This is not easy, but neither is it a cakewalk to live in constant pain. Choose to do what you have to do and do it now. As you recognize the multiple facets of your internal make-up you will naturally develop compassion for others and become more able to share and walk in their energies and they in yours.

As you work with your energy and discover new sources for it, you find that your attention broadens and your circle of interests enlarges. In your interpersonal interactions you will find your sensitivity to the plight of others increasing, and you will become more genuine and honest in expressing your needs, concerns, and ideas. The support for the old inner directed criticism will start to crumble and you will enjoy your own company and the company of others.

We all need to participate in our own healing. All of the patients I see in the course of a day are looking to others for help. They do need assistance, but improvement in quality of life will happen sooner if they take the attitude that there is more out there than meets the eye. We can all find new sources of energy in the wind, clouds, breath, and the words of others.

When it comes to these new ways of looking at our pain and frustrations it is important to remain open minded. Too many of us pride ourselves in being practical, but this attitude will maintain the blocks to healing. I had been seeing a middle-age man with a very early stage lung cancer. He had a cell type that was amendable to surgical resection. He did great with the surgery, as all of his cancer was removed. Follow up CAT scans and PET scans have remained negative, but he developed a post-thoracotomy syndrome. This is a painful condition that develops at the surgical site on the chest wall, leaving him with chronic pain since his surgery. He has tried multiple medical treatments including morphine, fentanyl, topical anesthetic patches and sprays, nerve ablation, and two trips to the acupuncturist.

On his last visit a week ago, I brought up the issue of beginning to look for the root cause of his persistent discomfort. After some discussion I handed him a photocopy of the directions for a "body scan" as described in Jon Kabat-Zinn's, *Full Catastrophe Living*.[6] His response was that he was too practical to practice with any seriousness.

In reviewing his condition, it appears that his continued pain may partially be the result of his underlying motivation. His brother-in-law was able to retire early on a medical disability and now has the time to do the things that he's always wanted to do. Maybe this gentleman's pain will ease once he gets disability, but in the meantime, over the past six to nine months he has been miserable.

In contrast to the gentleman above, I recently met a fellow beach lover who had a very positive experience with acupuncture therapy. He is a real estate agent who had suffered from problems in his rotator cuff (the four muscles that support the shoulder). He believes he initially injured it when he was seven or eight years old in the course of delivering daily newspapers. He also said he was a practical man, but had to admit that there was something to this "acupuncture thing" as it certainly helped him. This meeting was significant for me in that I too have sustained injury to my shoulder, and it was probably the result of carrying the morning papers in my paper-bag when I delivered papers as a kid. In keeping an open mind we find that we are not alone in our suffering, and realize that if one can overcome a painful condition, there is hope for all of us.

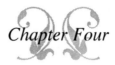

Chapter Four

Searching for Gold and Finding It

*M*oment by moment we continue on our individual quests just like the folks during the 1849 gold rush who packed up everything they owned, put it in a covered wagon, and headed west to find their fortunes. The gold we are searching for, held out in front of us like a lottery ticket, keeps us motivated and hoping that some day we will find the mother load. Television shows like "Who Wants to be a Millionaire?" so popular with Nielson ratings show a viewing audience of 36.1 million per episode in the United States alone, not to mention the millions of viewers in the 31 other countries in which it is aired. This alone confirms the notion that we all want to be rich and famous. Contestants on this syndicated game show are allowed to call on "lifelines," for help when they are not sure of an answer. Too many of us go through life without any internal lifelines and make decisions with only part of the information needed. We make life-changing decisions without fully understanding the consequences, or we continue on in the same vein day after day because of our own ignorance.

The insights gained from a meditation practice and the self-knowledge, acceptance, and new sources of energy harvested from yoga will help you develop and maintain such internal lifelines, making you more than a millionaire beyond financial terms. You will find riches within and experience more moments of contentment than ever before. There will be satisfaction no matter what is occurring in your life or in the lives of those you love.

If only we could be the next millionaires we could quit our jobs, buy new houses, invest the rest and live off the interest. The moment James Marshall discovered gold on Sutter's farm on January 28, 1848, Americans were no longer satisfied with the simple life. Everyone wanted to get rich quick.[1] When we are in pain we want a quick fix. Our minds start searching for a place where everything is perfect. We start deluding ourselves and make excuses as to why thing are the way they are and begin to ignore our own reality. This leads to more pain. We want to be worry free so the mind fools us into thinking that if we had all the money that we wanted, life would be trouble-free. We hold a mentality based on the magic of money when the real gold is to be found in the quiet mind, not a mind that is stressed, up against the wall, and cornered. If only we could afford to have someone else do our dishes and make our beds we would we free from pain.

The sad thing is that we are looking for our treasure in all the wrong places. A support group meets at our office once a month. It is a cozy gathering of surviving men and women coping with cancer. The underlying theme emerges as a healthy attitude toward life with all participants agreeing that they are living on borrowed time. They get up in the morning glad for the opportunity to experience what will come this day, finding pleasure and joy in simple things like mowing the lawn, planting and tending flowers and gardens, and sharing stories with each other on chemotherapy days. They now see each day as the gift that it is and their appreciation for what they have been given has multiplied in spite of and because of their cancer diagnosis.

We all want everything and we don't care to wait for it. Pushing ourselves to exhaustion we forget to seize the moment and enjoy ourselves. Instead we put all of our energy toward striving for the tangibles and have nothing left at the end of the day to celebrate the intangibles, like the unconditional love that our children show us, or the warm embrace of a supportive spouse. For those who suffer from painful conditions, pushing themselves continuously, there is no patience to make space for a few pain-free moments. The redeeming grace is that even those in chronic pain will get lost in the moment every now and then, but how many of these individuals are aware enough to know that they had just experienced a pain-free moment. Pain can consume us no matter where we stand financially.

In this next meditation we are going to seek the gold dust in our bodies and sprinkle it over those parts that give us the most pain. Attending to the breath as it hums in and out of the nasal passages, allow its rhythm to quell the rambling of the mind. As you find your quiet center, leisurely scan your body noticing where most of the pain is located. It may be behind or around the eyes, or in the neck, jaw, and shoulder area, or maybe in the lower back and legs. Wherever it is, be with it. As it grips you harder feel what muscle groups are doing the work of squeezing down.

Now rescan the body and find a place where you are currently pain-free. The only spot may be the fifth toe on your left foot, or your fingernail. In that precious place where there is no pain, savor that feeling. Examine and probe what it means to be without pain. This is the part of your physical body that is doing fine. It doesn't require your attention and is not calling out for any intervention on your part. Appreciate that sensation. What is there for you in this place of no need, in this place where you are resting? If you sense just empty space there ask yourself: how big is this space? Can you make it bigger by just thinking about it? Make it big enough to engulf your pain areas.

At this point you will begin to experience the "I," or ego, that will question your motives. The ego wants to know why you're taking your attention away from it. It has had your undivided attention and senses retreat and doesn't like it. Just listen to the internal dialogue as it happens for a moment then move on.

Now transfer your attention from this gold mine of painless existence and place the mind on an area of your body that has been a source of constant concern. Give your pain that new found space, knowing that there is more space where that came from. How do your attitudes differ between the two contrasting locations? See if you can allow yourself to incorporate a sense of health and well-being in both areas without looking at the troublesome area with a negative eye.

Let the sensations from the place of ease diffuse and insinuate into the area of distress. The human body is a complex organism that possesses unimaginable mechanisms for internal communication. The number of chemical messengers, hormones, enzymes, and cytokines that are floating around in our bodies are still being discovered. Just as when a patient receives chemotherapy for their cancer and the toxic chemicals work their way into the genetic makeup of the tumor cells thus rendering them incapable of reproduction, the good cells in the bone marrow are also affected. The result is a temporary drop in the white cells that normally help to fight infection, the red cells that carry oxygen to the tissues also decrease in numbers, and the platelets, the little cells that prevent bleeding, will fall. The body, sensing there has been a drop in counts, sends growth factors to the marrow, stimulating new growth of these much- needed cells.

In this way know that your mind and imagination have the same communicative capacities that upon your command will send the proper signals to the parts of your body that are in need of healing. This is just more of the gold within each of us; gold that we would never find it we did not begin prospecting. The early gold diggers dropped everything with the intention of finding what they were looking for. Most were not successful but the fact that they took the steps and started the journey forever changed their lives.

We have more control than we think we do when it comes to how we feel. Unfortunately we receive mixed messages being told it is not good to be a control freak. We obsess about our personal concerns and try to control that which is uncontrollable. In order to feel good about ourselves, it is necessary to stop giving our power away to thoughts and actions that have not borne fruit in the past. If coming from a place where family life was less than ideal or immersed in dysfunctional relationships, the move forward has to proceed with focus and undivided attention. Living in pain, you have learned to keep your mind on what bothers you and not on what feels good. In *Personality Characteristics of Patients With Pain* edited by Robert J. Gatchel, PhD. and James N. Weisberg, PhD., it is noted that optimism is an important mediator of stress and health.[2] There is growing recognition of the psychological and environmental factors associated with the interpretation of pain. Many individuals report significant pessimism when discussing their pain. Those trying to generate unrealistic optimism did not experience pain relief supporting the view that such patients preferred to focus on somatic or bodily complaints and ignored the suggestion that psychological factors also influence pain.

In the practice of yoga and meditation the goal becomes balance in everything. This includes looking at all of the factors that influence the manifestation of pain. Through movement of the body, in conjunction with intentional easing of the breath and relaxation of the mind, new ways of looking at situations reveal themselves. With time there will be many "ah-ha" moments. You begin to inquire more about "what if?" What if this pain is a message to change my outlook on life? What if I hold my head back more over my shoulders and allow the natural balance that follows to release chronic tension in the neck and jaws?

Even though personality characteristics are believed to be constant and unchangeable, this doesn't mean you have to continue looking at things as you always have. I saw a gentleman in the office last week with pancreatic cancer. He has done well, so far surviving over two years with the help of chemotherapy. We started talking about his home situation and dietary preferences as he was losing weight. He described how he does things at home and how he has always prepared his food in a particular way and that was just the way he was. As he spoke he appeared to physically harden. He was proud of the way he viewed himself and how he managed to care for himself, but he was stuck in that image even though his old ways were no longer serving him well. We all have places where we are stuck, where the energy is not moving because we have chosen, for whatever reason, to still the film and keep watching that one frame. Maybe we felt comfortable and the image had a soothing influence at the time so we held on to it. Fear of what was coming or fear of looking at another image of ourselves kept us in that place.

A little bit of pride is ok, but when pride gets us caught up in some past image of who we were and we continue to live from that image, it is no wonder that we find ourselves face to face with frustration. Awareness and recognition are the gold that we have to work with. If you truly want to see things with clarity, the way they really are, then you will. If you choose to stay where you are and not change any ideas of the self then at least be aware that this is what you are doing. Awareness is just like a muscle: the more you use it the stronger it will get, but we are also seeking flexibility. Being in tune with the rhythm of the breath gives us a constant point of focus that allows us to work on our awareness at any time.

At times we can't sleep and find ourselves awake in the middle of the night because of difficulties during the day or concerns about tomorrow. Take this opportunity to get in touch with the breath. Since you are already lying in bed, loosely stretch out on your back and place your arms at your sides with the palms facing up. Begin to notice and feel the breath moving in and out though the nostrils. Focus on the length of the breath. As you watch the breath, label each breath as a long breath or a short breath, depending on what you are finding at the moment. If you find the breath short and shallow you probably will not hear the breath as it enters and exits the body. At first you may not feel the rising and falling of the abdomen with each breath, but with time and increased awareness you will begin to notice these things. Along with this increasing awareness you will start to hear the hidden messages behind these breaths. Images of people in your life may arise. This is especially so of those who have had a significant impact in your life. This is the time to acknowledge their presence, thank them for what they have shown you and tell them goodbye. If you find that one or two images continue to come to mind then that person, or persons, have more than a healthy influence on you. Work is required to find out why you are holding on to them. It may be that at this time you lack full confidence in your own abilities to accomplish what it is that you need to for yourself, and are holding on to them for emotional support.

These images, though bothersome to you, are also gold nuggets to be mined. Their presence is a gift as you decided to hold on to them for support when you needed it. As you relied less and less on your own strength and wisdom to guide you, the images of others, at first thought to be helpful and soothing, have become your ghosts and tormentors. Now is the time to refine the gold and ask yourself just what it is that you want. What is it that will bring you happiness right now? What words do you need to hear from within that will bring you into harmony and balance? From this work you will hopefully fall off into a peaceful sleep.

Upon awakening the next morning, try a forward bend. The Sanskrit name for this asana is *uttanasana*. (See drawing or picture below). In this position you will find release and surrender. Allow the mind to fall into the lower body relaxing in the fullness of the bend. Just about everything we do is from an upright position. We get out of bed, stand and walk to the bathroom. Standing we bush our teeth then walk to the kitchen for breakfast. If we happen to drop something along the way we groan as we bend to pick it up, shake off the annoyance and move on. Finally when we go for our shoes, those of us who have laces will have to bend over to tie them. With the invention of loafers we don't have to bother bending. The main reason remaining for bend-ing over seems to be to pick something up.

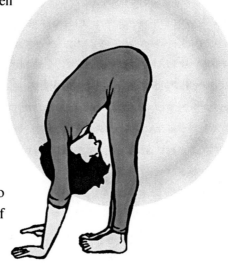

Forward Bend

In a forward bend we allow the muscles of the lower back to stretch and lengthen. In our constant upright position the large paraspinal muscles that run bilaterally along the length of the spine have a tendency to pull in on themselves and tighten. The result is a chronic nagging pain that seems to never go away. While in the position of a forward bend we can relax as the breath broadens the muscles of the lower back and torso. In this position we notice that the breath entering the belly will massage the upper thighs, help-ing over time to make them supple, thus giving them more internal space.

The beauty of having a basic knowledge of yoga is that you can call upon it at any time to give your mind and body just what they are calling for. In the middle of the day, while at work or home, when tightness in the neck makes itself known you can sneak away and do a forward bend. Let the weight of the head deepen the bend while extending the arms to the floor if possible. If you are unable to reach the floor with your hands then rest them on your thighs. Breathe and allow the inner tension and the movement of the breath to massage the body. Upon standing you will notice a new awareness. You will be cognizant of your next breaths and will feel more present than you had before.

This is all just more precious metal that you are given to work with. The increasing awareness that you develop over time will help you to recognize at an earlier moment when you are beginning to tense up. Tension is just wasted energy keeping you in a state of hyper- alertness. This inappropriate tension takes us out of the natural rhythm and throws us off kilter like extra atrial beats of the heart when we drink too much caffeine. Effectiveness is optimized when we are in balance. A forward bend takes a minimal amount of effort and requires just a bit of balance and concentration. It takes an attitude of letting go to perform a forward bend, so this position helps us learn to expend less effort in getting what we want. How many things in life are you trying to achieve from this perspective? Usually we have to concentrate, push, force, and cajole to get what we want. Why not take the time to just give in and slip into a forward bend. It will cool your internal heat and slow things down enough for you to get a better idea of what is happening internally.

Many patients complain of having weakness in the legs and hips. When receptive I will show them simple movements they can perform any time while sitting comfortably in a chair. If they happen to require a wheelchair they can practice from there. Remember any movement is better than no movement. Movement performed without awareness; rote and done out of habit, keeps us locked in old unproductive, painful ways.

It is difficult to find gold in the midst of suffering. There will always be something to worry about if that is your modus operandi. Even the most successful individuals have problems, but they turn their problems into nuggets of gold helping them attain what they seek. When we welcome problems and look at them as a means of gaining experience and proficiency then we can go about our business without being thrown by every big wave that comes our way.

If we can look at our suffering and acknowledge it then we can begin to cultivate a "so what" attitude that will take the punch out of pain. The pain may persist but the suffering will not be as intense. This concept is easy to describe and just as easy to reject on the grounds that is sounds ridiculous and unproductive. It takes minute by minute wakefulness to live this way and is so much better than the alternative of living with suffering. We already know what that is like. Negative feelings and ideas are going to arise but they do not need to have power over us. They take power from us when we choose to focus on them. Once we make the decision to shift our attention to the moment, the energy conserved is employable towards endeavors that bring contentment.

Our words are our gold. We attract what we vocalize. When we say, "that's just the way I am," we have chosen to settle for our limited ideas of the self. We have essentially said that, "I can't possibly do that because I have never tried." When we stay open to new opportunities the freshness of our minds will tell us what the next step needs to be.

It is easier to look at our neighbors and compare our lives to theirs than it is to examine our own lives. When we can be happy over the success of those in our circles then we remain open to the free flow of bounty to us. Helen is a lady who works in our office. Her role is to assist patients and their families who are in need. The needs are usually financial, but other times there are emotional and social needs. Helen is a cancer survivor of almost twenty years. She, like the rest of us, has not been without tribulation. In the prime of life her niece and her niece's husband were killed in an automobile accident. Helen's way of remembering them has been through giving.

Her giving has culminated in the establishment of a foundation called, Pennies From Angels. Donors bring in their pennies and Helen distributes the monies to those with the greatest need. Pennies From Angels has helped patients buy medicines, pay their heating bills, purchase gasoline, and even buy Christmas presents for children who otherwise would do without. When there is a major function for cancer survivors Helen canvasses local businesses for financial support and usually gets it in the form of donated food. There is nothing Helen would rather do than help others. In all of her endeavors she has the assistance and support of her husband Cliff, as they both share in the giving of their love and talents. The knowledge that they are helping those in need is their gold.

When we choose to do something from the heart word gets around. People come from out of no where to help. In Helen's work she is always amazed at the help she receives. Many times she hasn't a clue as to how things are going turn out, but as she follows her impulses those on the receiving end always end up with more than they anticipated. Her reputation has grown as a patient advocate. For the past two years she has been invited to Washington, DC to educate our lawmakers about the day to day needs of cancer patients, especially those in rural America. She is a lady that looks for gold in everything and usually finds it, thus benefiting everyone.

Using picks and shovels gold miners sifted through tons of sand, dirt, and rock to get to the gold. Today, to mine our inner gold, our tools are the imagination, our intention, and our breath. With effort and concentration we can rearrange skewed anatomy and restore symmetry to our muscles even after years of misuse and wrong thought. The rock walls of thought surrounding our hurts can be broken down, but we don't want to use explosives tearing everything up in the process. The key is to start this process with gentleness yet also maintain a firm conviction that you will find balance. It is just like the ocean waves that move the sand with each pulse, continually changing the landscape.

Like anything else of value, the techniques taught here will not be grasped in one sitting. It will take repeated trials and readjustments of the mind and muscles to bring everything back to balance. One of the most difficult things to do is to just let go. We wake up every day and defend our ideas of who we think we are. We pick and choose what to focus on all day long based on our beliefs and preferences. We spend so much time trying to figure out how to do something instead of just doing it. When we move into doing what we want to we learn as we go, viewing mistakes as part of the learning process and not as a reason to tell ourselves that there is something wrong with us. It is all in the attitude. Why not just stop being so hard on ourselves and start doing what is comfortable. There are a finite number of "have to's" that need to get done everyday, but after that the rest of the time is open for us to do what we want. If you are at a place where your not sure of what would make you happy then this is a perfect time to begin your meditation practice.

In your quiet place start by suggesting to yourself that you are going to come up with some ideas of what you would like to experience in your life. This is not to be confused with what you have to do to pay the rent or mortgage, but what you think you would enjoy doing. It may be something as far out as skidooing off the shores of Cancun. Getting into your quiet space and following the breath to your center begin to smell the salt water. Feel the heat on your skin as the sun soaks you to your core. Hear the roar of the motor as you twist the throttle. As the splashing water makes your tanned skin glisten it cools your chest. You are there because you want to be. You can keep coming back to this place to enjoy the rewards of your imagination.

As you sit, the next question needs to be how do you get to this place in real time? What steps will it take? It might mean working some overtime to pay for the trip. It might mean looking into travel bargains on the Internet or it may be as simple as calling your travel agent. Eventually you will find yourself in Cancun. So it is with yoga and meditation. As you ask yourself what will it take to be pain free, and what will it take to have greater balance in life you will be shown which direction to take to make this happen. It is all a matter of where we focus our attention. The early pioneers and gold seekers had no idea what they were getting into. They heard stories, good and bad, about what had happened to others before them, but when things got bad enough where they were they decided to move out and take the chance. We are in the same place. We either choose to keep things the way they are and live with it, or we make up our minds to change things and move into unknown territory. Going to this place forces us to look at our situations from a different perspective and fosters creative thinking in that we are no longer functioning from habitual patterns.

The paradox in all of this is that once we are able to accept things the way they are then we are ripe for change and things do change. When we can continually ask ourselves, how can we do this better and tell ourselves there must be an easier way then we know that we are making our own way.

Our families are another part of our gold mine in that they are the gems that keep us on our toes. Those of us with young children are in the best position to learn with every encounter. Children are honest because they know no other way. Too many of us go around fooling ourselves and thinking that we are fooling others. Afraid of seeing the truth we color our lives the way we ideally want them to be when in reality we are creating more substrate for pain and suffering. One day we may wake up and realize that we suffered more than we had too because we did not trust that we would receive what we needed. Living our lives to please others is just another way to say hit me. Others may not actually strike at you but you are beating yourself up for not taking care of your needs. When we truly listen to our children and allow them to express their feelings without interjecting what we think they should be feeling then we will learn the meaning of allowing others to be themselves. Once we can do this then we can work to become what we truly want to be. When we wake up in the morning and have our first thoughts be that today I am going to be kind to my children then we can be assured that we will treat ourselves with the same kindness. Too many of us are hard on ourselves, pushing and forcing to do things that we may not enjoy just to live a certain lifestyle or to drive a particular kind of car. Twenty-four carrot gold is soft and not hard like the gold bricks we see the bad guys trying to steal in the movies. So until we can soften to ourselves we will pay the price of continued pain and we won't even know why we are hurting.

The same holds true for listening. In order to truly listen to someone we have to tell ourselves that we are going to listen, otherwise we will continue on with our own internal conversation and not understand fully what the other's message is. The fact that most of us are not good listeners is no surprise. There is too much going on all around us and it's all vying for our attention. Our body is yelling at us to change the way we do and see things by causing us pain. The more we ignore the message the more intense and unrelenting the pain becomes. What is it going to take to get us to listen? Why not start doing the yoga and the meditation so that at least the mind and the body have a chance to get on the same page. In this next exercise I would like for you to get into your quiet place and imagine that you are going to have a conversation with the one person that you truly respect and admire. Call this person your hero if you would like to. As you follow your breathing and move inside allow this inner space to expand. Imagine yourself sitting face to face with this person whom you admire. Instead of telling your story in detail, allow this witness and helper to undergo the same trials that you have been going through. See that person's facial expression, feel their mood, listen for their words as they talk to you about the challenges ahead of them. You may find that your "hero" doesn't even entertain the idea of failure, when this is all that you have been focusing on. Seeing yourself back in your situation you may be frowning, or anxious, or on the verge of tears, while your supporter may be as relaxed as ever. We all have different backgrounds and when we have lived through trauma our nervous systems become and stay more revved up than they should. This leads to chronic anxiety even over things that are non-threatening to others. Allow yourself to accept the attitude of those you respect and make them your own. It will require that you put your own ego aside for a while and for some of us that is the most difficult thing to do. Yoga and meditation will show you how to incorporate these attitudes into your daily life as you discover that your life and your story are your gold. We have to trust, work, dig, and sweat to reach our full potential. Don't settle for less.

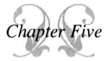

Chapter Five

Fire Plus O_2 → A New You

*C*an you feel your fire, the energy that motivates you? Or are you impeding your own progress by snuffing the flames of passion in your life? Afraid of our own power, squelching the inner voice that tells us to do it, to try it and go for it, we propagate our pain and depression. We either practice to make strides ahead or our ingrained actions cause us persistent frustration. There are things we can do to feel more alive right now. The visions that we hold, now dim, of what our lives would look and feel like if we were living to our full potential are meant to be expressed. It is time to revisit the attitudes and beliefs that are holding us back.

There are secondary gains achieved by persisting in current thinking. In order to move on it is necessary to do some difficult work. It is difficult in the sense that we are comfortable living the way we do, even though we are empty. To get out of the box and feel the refreshing breeze takes courage, but that is not a problem, since we have plenty of courage, as we have been living with suffering for so long.

Life will open up when we dare to change our thinking. Fear is an issue, but by looking at fear we gain power to make things happen by understanding that fear is empty. It has power over us only to the degree that we allow. To take responsibility for what happens in our lives we must stand up for what we believe in and begin to let others know what we need.

To stoke our fires and have life move like fire fanned by the howling winds we find ourselves more awake. Fear of getting burned and afraid to lose what we already have impairs our ability to heal. Opening our hearts frees us to give up the worn out ideas that we have been living for years. This opens and clears the way to receive the manifestation of our dreams. Our fire can move us to seriously try to make something positive happen.

What others say or think is not an issue. Our wisdom goes deeper than the limits of others, but we have to be open to hear it. It is good to know fear. There are real fears in the world. Fear keeps us from doing harmful things but ungrounded fear will hold us back from the enjoyment we seek and crave. Sitting down and listing some of our unreal fears we give ourselves the chance to see our worst nightmares. We have the ability to go to bed at night and direct our minds to confront these dragons and in the same night lay the groundwork to conquer these enemies within. It is possible because we are in charge of our dreams. Every part of the dream is a part of us. Make it what you what and don't let your fear draw the negative to you.

We are also in charge of what we experience during our waking hours. We determine how we react to everything that happens to us. There are issues in our past that we would like to forget but just can't let go of. We have beliefs about ourselves that prevent us from changing and reinventing ourselves. We have to be willing to drop beliefs that we are lazy or forgetful, or that we were destined to live in pain.

The first step in changing our mind is to make the clear intention that we have all that it takes to light our fires. Living in our dualistic state with likes, dislikes, preferences, and opinions we have lost sight of the clarity of our nature. We have, as Tenzin Wangyal Rinpoche explains in *The Tibetan Yogas of Dream and Sleep*, lost our ability to have direct experience.[1] We taint everything that we see and experience with our beliefs and expectations. Are you willing to drop old ideas that haven't worked for you in the past and move on to what is really happening now? If so, you will live in the moment facing trials, problems, and challenges and feel more alive than you ever had.

The fear of fire is a very healthy fear. To know this as fear is to live realistically. The Minnesota Multiphasic Personality Inventory is a psychological test developed by Hathaway and McKinley in 1943.[2] Life experience paradigms are presented that assess personality traits such as self-confidence, anxiety, fear, and depression. The older test has been supplanted by the MMPI-2. Besides it's usefulness in the diagnosis of mental disorders, it has utility in assessing and developing treatment strategies for patients with chronic pain. The MMPI-2 has been useful in helping to determine how "comfortable" a patient with chronic pain is in their sick role.[3] There are multiple scales within the MMPI-2 that have indicated that there are common features exhibited by patients who suffer from chronic pain. These individuals tend to score high on scales representing hypochondriasis, indicating a readiness on their part to exhibit pain behaviors. They may also have high scores on the depression and hysteria scales. Those with high scores on the depression scale experience a great deal of distress over their painful conditions were as those with low scores indicated a low cost, or low distress related to their pain conditions.

In *The Zen Path Through Depression*, Philip Martin tells us the following:

> "In depression we experience intense pain that is both physical and mental. We also frequently complicate that pain through our attempts to get away from it. And often we are unaware of just how much we are suffering, because we are so involved in trying to outrun our pain, or ignore it, or cover it up with anger." [4]

Most of us have a worst time of day. With some effort, that time can be pinpointed, and inquiry can be made into the root of these feelings. What scenes come to mind? What feelings flood into consciousness? What muscles tighten up, especially around the neck, throat, and shoulders to invite greater anxiety? What brings on relaxation and resolution? If you have pain, you have anger. If you have anger then you have fire. It behooves us to become aware of the time of day when we are at our worst or at the point of intolerance to our pain. This is where we will find our fire. The embers may be barely lit as they were in the children's story, the *Little Engine That Could*, just after the engine was buried by the avalanche at the summit on it's way to deliver toys to the children. Determination and support from his friends kept that tank engine's fire alive. It will take determination, intention, faith, effort, and support from others to break through our pain conditions, but we must be willing and ready to look at our anger and deal with it.

Meditation offers the arena for seeing the anger clearly while yoga offers the playing field for burning it off without bringing harm to others or ourselves.

When we are lost in anger and the fire is burning out of control we find there is a total lack of internal communication. You know you are angry and you are consumed by this state of mind to the point that nothing else can get in. By following our breath and observing it moving in and out of the lungs we can redirect the energy of anger and diffuse our own pain. Mastery will not occur overnight but with even the slightest improvement in your skill to manage the anger you will appreciate the power gleaned from this forceful emotion.

Thich Nhat Hanh in his book, *Anger: Wisdom for Cooling the Flames*, offers suggestions for looking at your anger more deeply. He recommends that the moment you discover your mind engulfed with anger that you intentionally tell yourself the following: "Seeing myself burned by the fire of anger, I breathe in. Feeling compassion for myself burning with anger, I breathe out." Normally we continue holding on to our anger until we feel that we have finally had our way. We wait until the other person gives in to us or until they make a move to appease us. As long as we remain in our conditioned state and as long as others allow this behavior to persist there will be no motivation to change. The awareness to begin understanding the pathways our anger takes to manifestation has to come from within. There has to be a burning desire to want to understand the why in our anger response and the internal tape has to be interrupted in order to be changed.

When the fire of anger is raging within what pictures are you seeing in your mind? Whose words are you listening to? There is a root to your anger as there is a root to everything that you believe and do. Allow the breath to perform the microdissection for you. Use it to slow the mind and quell the flames then take the energy of the anger to formulate the response that you want from a place of mindfulness. In the back of your mind you hold a picture of the person that you want to be. Now is the time to work to bring that image into daily manifestation. Begin to ask yourself each time you feel your anger rising who is experiencing this anger? Asking this question enough times will show you the answer. The wonderful thing about the answer is that there is no right answer, it is not static, and it is constantly changing as you change.

A great exercise to perform, which will assist us in manifesting our dreams, is to sit down and write out the events and expectations of a perfect day, listing each experience hour by hour. While you are at it take the time to review your past responses to anger provoking situations. In one column write down how you typically react with your anger and in another column jot down how you would like to mindfully respond to a situation that causes you anger. It is healthy to express your anger when it is done from your center while it only makes you more emotional if you react with outbursts. You will be heard when you respond from the center and you will be ignored when anger has taken your senses away.

Fear and anger go hand in hand. Are you afraid of being here? Natalie Goldberg says in her CD titled, *Zen Howl*, that we constantly allow thoughts to flood our minds because of a fear of being here. Being here is too real. It used to make her heart race. For some people they need to get their hearts jump started. For too long they have let life meander by, afraid of getting their hearts racing over anything. I remember as a medical student how my heart felt like it was going to rip out of my chest because of fear prior to giving a presentation. With sweaty palms, my thoughts would accelerate to a speed that was draining. All of this happened because of anxiety over talking in front of a group. Over the years I have observed doctors and medical students give successful and enjoyable talks. I have also suffered though some talks that were so poorly thought out and so uninspiring that it was painful to sit there and watch the presenter flounder. Over time I learned that the racing heart could just as easily be labeled excitement instead of fear. By labeling the feeling as excitement the prospect of giving a talk became a source of fun and pleasure. It became an opportunity to share knowledge with others. It helped to realize that not everyone would agree on all of the content but overall the audience walked away feeling that their time had been well spent.

Why remain afraid of the pounding in the chest? Take a deep breath. Don't live life so close to the inner safety net, that the lungs begin to collapse on themselves, thus limiting the life force from entering and moving you. We can view oxygen as the fuel of life. The air we breathe is the high octane of our inner engines that we have been blessed with for the short time we are here. Look at individuals who suffer with emphysema. They have to intentionally move slowly and deliberately. They have no choice. Their muscles cannot function adequately because their lungs cannot deliver the oxygen that is physiologically needed.

Air is free. It may not always be as clean as we want, but it is there for us to use as we wish. Breathe deeply and take in all that is meant to be yours. On the exhalation let everything go. Drop it. Poof! It's gone. It is no longer yours. It has vaporized and you are relaxed, yet energized. The breath is your chisel. The breath will mold and shape you into your best self. By consciously following your breath healing takes place. By allowing the breath do what it is supposed to we reclaim our lives. We need to get out of our own way.

Focusing on and working with the energy of our breath or *pranayama* is the fourth of the eight limbs of yoga as described in the *Yoga Sutras of Patanjali*.[v] The other stages or limbs are the following: 1) *yama* (abstinence), 2) *niyama* (observance), 3) *asana* (posture), 5) *pratyahara* (sense withdrawal), 6) *dharana* (concentration), 7) *dhyana* (meditation), and 8) *samadhi* (contemplation, absorption or superconscious state). Through awareness of the breath we become aware of the body. Most joggers, swimmers, and exercise buffs are very proficient at taking their pulses. On the other hand the rest of the population, those not in the medical profession, lack knowledge on how to take a pulse. Unfamiliar with the location of the radial artery in the lateral aspect of the wrist, where the radius meets the metacarpal bones, most folks never had the need nor bothered to learn how to monitor their cardiac performance. Thanks to the movies most Americans have heard and know of the carotid arteries in the neck, but few have ever taken the time or had the instruction on how to actually take a pulse there. With a normal heart rate in the range of 60 – 100 beats per minute it is very difficult to monitor the heart rate with any accuracy and consistency over time.

The respiratory rate and the pattern of the breath are much more accessible bodily functions to follow. Just like the heartbeat our breath is ever present. Ask anyone who suffers from asthma or emphysema how anxious it makes them feel not to be able to catch their breath. When all efforts are directed toward securing the next breath there is not much energy left to invest in life's little pleasures. This is also the case for those who suffer from chronic pain or emotional pain associated with major life changes. Divorce, job dissatisfaction, financial concerns, moving into a new dwelling, or facing the multitude of frustrations that are evident for those with the mindset of just going along to tolerate life are situations common to many and unless acted upon in a constructive way these events deplete the life energy.

Since the breath is always with us it can be used as a barometer and a rudder. The quality of the breath will tell the practitioner the degree of anxiety that is present. By observing the breath moving through the body you can also feel where your muscles are holding on. In a tight spot, such as the neck, with attention you will know where the flow is impeded. There will be a squeezing tightness with associated burning heat. Unfortunately the longer this tightness is ignored the more difficult it is to release it because of the associated muscle contractures and binding of the myofascia. As mentioned earlier, calcium will eventually deposit in these areas, blood flow will be decreased, and neuropraxia or nerve dullness will ensue.

To get over the pain you have to be willing to look at the pain. It literally hurts and that is why everyone wants to take a pill to fix it but there are no such pills. There are products from nature that are used in medicine all of the time. Digitalis, a drug used to treat heart failure originally came from the leaves of the foxglove plant *digitalis lanata*. Like everything in life, you can get too much of a good thing and too much digitalis will slow the heart to the point of asystole leading to cardiac arrest. The chemotherapeutic agent Taxol, originally used to treat ovarian cancer and now also used to treat breast, lung, head and neck, and bladder cancers also came directly out of the forest. It was discovered in the stem bark of the Pacific Yew tree, *Taxus brevifolia* in 1967. The trees grow only in the northwest Pacific coastal region of the United States.

Reading this you may think that this is too easy or that something as "simple" as the breath can't possibly have that much power and potential. Stop for a moment and think back to the last time you gazed upon the ocean.

Standing on the shore you could see the varying height of the waves as they melodiously undulated toward the shore. You heard their movement as they spilled over on themselves and each other. From this vantage point you sensed a hint of their power but to truly experience their impact you had to get into the water, at least waist high, and get tossed around and pushed over to really feel their power. It felt good to resist the oncoming flow until a larger wave came along and lifted you off your feet depositing you on shore with shell-torn knees and elbows. This is the same power that the breath possesses. Until you get into the study and practice of working with your breath there is no way you can come to realize what it can do for you.

Many are of the mindset that if you don't have to pay for something then it has no worth. Everyday we hear, "You get what you pay for." This is true when it comes to buying a new car where the heated leather seats, the four-wheel drive, and the variable speed wipers on the newest SUV are going to cost much more than the rubber mats and cloth seats of a Honda Element. It is also true when it comes to buying a house in that the more money you spend the more elaborate, decorative, and hopefully, durable the house will be. When it comes to inner truth, taking away all of the externals, there is still a price to pay but it is not monetary. The price is your time, commitment, and your faith. Are you willing to invest in yourself and witness a reawakening?

If you have so much pain that you don't know where else to turn, what have you to lose by spending some time with yourself and your breath. Let the breath be your guide. Let it be the wave that brings new hope and new life to you. Let it cut through all of the old stuff you've been holding on to and allow it to renew your being. Stop telling yourself that you can't do anything about your situation and stop ignoring the gifts of your breath, mind, body, and spirit.

With this next exercise the goal is to find your smooth even breath. When you were a child and did not get your way your only resort was to cry. With an outburst of tears and sobs your body jerked and your speech stuttered as you tired to get your needs and desires known. Like a Craftsman ratchet your breath would start-stop, start-stop as you cut it off with your emotion. Mindfully extending your arm at the elbow you can feel the smooth, even working muscles carry out the command of your mind. On the other hand when a patient with Parkinson's disease moves their arm they experience a phenomena that is best described as gegenhalten or counter-pull. This is a condition of involuntary resistance to movement of the extremities. As more pressure is applied to moving the arm a greater resistance to movement ensues. When you are tense and anxious the same events occur with your breath and you limit the energy available to you.

In other words, the more you try the greater resistance you come up against. You need to be willing to let go, drop any ideas of who you think you are and stay open to the sensations and visions that arise.

When asking your muscles to lift something beyond their limit they shake, tremble, and vibrate from overexertion. Eventually the muscles fatigue and the object falls to the ground. In this exercise you will be looking for areas of tightness in your respiratory apparatus that may unknowingly be binding your breath. Any tension that restricts the movement of the diaphragm, or limits the even expansion and contraction of the intercostal muscles (the muscles between your ribs) will also arrest the breath. If you are sitting in a slumped position the weight of the body will also inhibit the free movement of the respiratory muscles. In addition, any unnecessary tension that is maintained in the head and neck areas will impede the free flow of the life breath.

Find your quiet place and position yourself so that you maintain an erect back. Intend to accentuate the normal lordotic curve of the lumbar spine. Bring your pelvis forward so that you are sitting on the "sit bones" of the bottom of the pelvis.

You may find it easier at first to sit on a four to six inch high pillow. This will help bring your pelvis forward. Begin by feeling the movement of each breath as it enters the nose. Feel the contact that the flow of oxygen makes

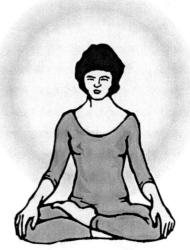

Proper sitting position

with the nasal mucosa (the inner lining of the nose). For the entire length of your respiratory cycle, with each inspiration and expiration, keep your focus on the movement of air as it courses through the nasal passage. As you notice your attention moving away from the point of concentration, gently bring your mind back to the breath as it bathes the nasal mucosa. You will notice your mind starting to wander and will change your point of focus many times, but each time come back to the breath. Things you have to do will come to mind. Do not react to any of these thoughts; simply come back to the breath. Visions of past events will arise, notice them and bring the attention back. Worries and concerns will surface. Let them go. As you continue following the breath, begin to experience your own presence. Frequent practice with this method will help you discriminate between your imaginary inner battles and the real challenges that face you. Through persistent work with the breath you will discover what steps you need to take to move into greater balance. When we stop trying for force things to happen and begin to visualize, and work with intention, things start to change. To be able to function in such a way in all areas of our lives brings new hope for the concept of effortless living. Imagine having energy to spare at the end of the day to play with the kids, to have meaningful conservation with our significant other, to read and ponder. Begin to sense that the flames of the fire within are ready to roar again.

Thinking back we can determine who or what put our fires out. At some crucial point a decision was made to quell our flames, but since making the decision the reasons are long repressed. By summoning our inner courage we can explore to determine what events or inner dialogue led us to douse our energy source. It may have been a look, a word, or a feeling that we were too young to understand that led us to making the decision to withdrawal. With the proper intention and the calming, quieting effects of an easy breath, we can stay with these thoughts long enough, even through the pain we are feeling, to find a spark of truth. With time, patience, and perseverance the inner truth will unfold. As we listen we may hear the voices of others but what is needed is courage to go beyond that to hear what is deeper and true for you. Are there any insights that want to surface? If there are, stay with the feeling and follow the impulse.

During these explorations do not be impulsive. Give yourself time to process all of the new incoming information. When you buy a new car you don't just go out and purchase the first one you see. First you think about the reasons why you want the car. Usually a discussion with a significant other follows. The financial implications and practical uses for the car are reviewed. The resale value, interest rates, and maintenance records for the particular vehicle are considered. When you are ready then you buy the car.

When it comes to dealing with our hidden emotions and underlying motivations it is useful to forget about what is practical and just go with gut feeling. This is the time to look beyond the superficial, deeper than the external façade, and into the realm of the soul's movements. If your attention is always directed outward there is less chance of fueling your own fire from within. It can be fruitful to follow that line of reasoning and go beyond where the mind goes. You can bring your deepest desires to fruition and overcome your mental, physical, and emotional pain by staying awake to what moves you and acting on these internal directions. The energy for all of this work is now tied up in your pain. Begin to ponder what life would be like without your pain and start to contemplate how you are going to finally give up your pain forever.

The pain may keep coming back to one place or region day after day. It is still the fire - use it. Do not let it consume you and overwhelm you. Your breath and your body are intimately connected so use the breath to free the body and free the blocked energy that is causing your pain. It is possible to extricate yourself from your rut but you need to pay attention to the breath and not be afraid of the fire. It is the flame that brings us to places not predicted. It takes the boredom out of daily existence and allows for life's potential to fill each of us. Life is meant for us to live. It is not something that the other person experiences but what we can all experience to a fuller degree when we let things unfold naturally without resistance. Let the fire burn!

We limit our experiences by going into situations thinking that we know the outcome. We tell ourselves that we will go to work everyday and put up our walls tolerating the same continual frustrations. It is the same old thing day after day. It will turn out like we expect it to. The same thing holds for our attitudes about our pain. By telling ourselves that we will never be rid of the pain, it has no choice but to stay. It is fine to admit to yourself that you have no clue on how to remove yourself from this condition, but then ask the necessary next question with following the breath: What ideas, attitudes, and beliefs do I need to get rid of to be free from my pain? The answer will come if you persist and the universe will bring new experiences your way. The power in life seems to express itself when we get out of its way. When we try to control things and events our human nature limits us and we unknowingly limit our experience.

What kind of food fuels our energy systems? When we take time at night to read something that is meaningful, the next day those thoughts and concepts find a way into our day. Prior to falling off to sleep it is helpful to again follow your breath. Begin by taking long easy breaths, allowing the thoracic cavity to fill smoothly without tension. The character of the long breath is restful. When taking this breath in silently count 1-2-3-4. At the end of the inspiration hold the breath, without fighting it, again for a count of four: 1-2-3-4. Then slowly and smoothly allow the breath to naturally seep out of the lungs as follows: 1-2-3-4-5-6-7-8. Rest for a count of two and repeat until centered and calm.

Yoga and meditation can lead you to a place where you can discharge pent up harmful emotions without causing any harm to yourself or others. They are powerful tools to have at your disposal. When anger tries to consume you the skills necessary to deal with it effectively will be within reach. Reading about this emotion in Thich Nhat Hanh's book, *Anger*, he refers to his loved one's on this physical plane, as well as his thoughts, as "darlings." He sees his anger as being like a child who needs kind attention and gentle handling. After reading his passages, I find that I refer to my own thoughts as darlings the next day without effort. He shows us a new, fresh, and healthy way to look at our anger. His instruction to us is to speak to our loved one first in our imaginations then go to them with an understanding voice saying that we did not mean to hurt them, that we love them, and want the best for them and our relationship. He asks the loved one to teach him and help him to love. It is not a plea. It is not being subservient. It is being genuine. We can do this same thing and direct it toward the self within that we dislike, the self that is allowing us to continue on with our pain.

Wanting to express love, it will come across. There is no hiding it when we make a connection on a deeper level. As we speak to our loved one with gentleness and kindness so we can speak to ourselves. It is so important when working with our own difficult issues and emotions to be gentle. As Richard Freeman tells us in *Yoga Breathing*, we need to approach this difficult work wearing an inner smile. The last thing we want to do is to beat ourselves up.

When we first go to light a fire, be it at a campsite or at home on a cold winter night, we do not throw the heavy logs directly onto the kindling. We know to wait until the fire gets hotter and bigger. If we tried to put the heavy logs on the fire too early the fire goes out. The same thing holds when working with our difficult emotions. We have to first tease them out of their hiding places. We have to give them space. We have to acknowledge our feelings without criticism; otherwise they will go back into hiding and continue to bother us. Let the oxygen feed the fire and let's not allow the heavy logs to smother out the life of the fire. In the same way, being gentle with ourselves we do not stir up the anger, which is the fire-packed emotion. Anger needs to be acknowledged before it can be transformed into compassion by understanding.

Our thoughts can either be more kindling for the fire or act as water for the fire. It depends on what we tell ourselves. It takes a mind that is willing to pay attention to the continual inner dialogue and a mind that is willing to question everything that goes on within. It is OK to be lazy in the sense of allowing sometime for relaxation. On the other hand it is not useful to be lazy in the sense that we shy away from policing our own thoughts. We can not afford to let our minds go everywhere they want just as we cannot let our children watch as much TV as they want. Neither can we allow them to stay up as late as they want to. There is a price to pay for such laxity and the price is suffering.

Fire needs oxygen. Without it fire does not have the right conditions to exist. Can you find a way to listen to your breath at moments when you typically start to get angry or upset, at moments when you begin to feel that issues are starting to get hooked by someone else's words or behavior? Let the breath be the guide. Allowing the breath to open us completely we are able to see what it is that we are doing. Let the breath be the gateway to increased awareness. As the breath begins to tease the fire into existence and the fire begins to flare do not be afraid of the energy. Look for ways to use the fire for inner transformation.

Get to the center with the fire and discover it is not something separate from you. You are one with it. The fire will separate the ore from the gold and will do so only if we allow it to. It takes courage to look at our own stuff. Years and years of habits will go away if we choose not to ignore them and look for their roots. Realize that it will take great patience to do this work on a consistent basis. Extend the patience typically given to a newborn baby. In everyone's eyes a newborn is innocent and has done no wrong. Pure and untouched by the ways and thoughts of the world, you are that baby and possess such innocence. It takes a soft touch and an open mind. It takes a mind that is willing to put the big adult self on the shelf and let that baby be. Watch the self talk here as all sorts of criticism will try to stop these efforts. Know that it is a way that ego is using to regain control.

There is no need to be controlled by anyone or anything. We can exist in pure form at all times without having to fit into one type of mold or another. Become fluid. Become soft. Get gentle. Get open. Look and see what is happening. There is a quiet within that we ignore. It resides within us but in our desire to avoid our inner worlds we are always looking for something on the outside to fulfill us. Any little noise is allowed to hold our attention. Can we not sit in front of the crackling fire, feel it's warmth, be soothed by it's glow, and yet be still in the presence of the embers? In the same way we can center ourselves from the inside and be aware of what is happening around us. We do not have to be taken away by such activity. When we are able to center we can be more fully present and in being so we become more effective. Let the fire burn without the fear of consumption.

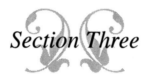

Section Three

CHOOSING
THE
MIDDLE PATH

Section Three

CHOOSING THE MIDDLE PATH

Introduction

*I*n today's world everyone and everything seems to be moving to
extremes. With extreme skateboarding, biking, and motorcycle compe-
titions, individuals risk life and limb to gain the top spots and revel in the
limelight. Top corporations expect extreme sacrifices from their employees
and demand "team players" to put self and family second behind the quest
for the highest market share and profits. An individual's value has been
sadly shifted from intrinsic worth to how much income he can generate.
These are not just modern day concerns but seem to be more extreme today.
In 1785 Immanuel Kant wrote of behaving morally toward others with
respect for the individual and not what that individual could do for you.[1]
John F. Kennedy reiterated this need to get away from a taking attitude to
one of helping others in his Inaugural Address of January 20, 1961 when he
spoke, "And so, my fellow Americans: ask not what your country can do for
you – ask what you can do for your country."

With each decision we make there is a choice and a freedom to choose
the middle path. Awareness of this fact brings with it individual power and
self- responsibility. By daily tapping into our internal wisdom it is possible
to truly know thyself. The drive and push to overachieve and work until
exhaustion, in an effort to gain respect and approval, will be replaced by
knowledge of one's own intrinsic value. Knowing when to drop your story

line and just be present will lead to greater moments of joy and less pain and aggravation. That these negative emotional states are self-induced is often forgotten.

Through the practices of surrender and acceptance you will free up great quantities of energy. This energy can be used to bring your life into greater balance on a more consistent basis. To live a healthy life it is necessary to strive for balance though it is not always easy to balance work with play, individual time with family or group time, or sleep and rest with activity. This is especially difficult if you are dealing with chronic pain of any etiology.

To find balance many of us must first lighten up and relax. We have to let go of much of our self- induced expectations and pretensions. A willingness to sit in meditation and commit yourself to staying with whatever comes up is the first step to take in bringing balance and freedom. You will find with practice that it is possible to relax even in the presence of your pain and tribulations.

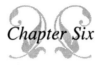

Chapter Six

More Than a Physical Body: Can You Feel It?

*W*e go through life with specific ideas of who we are, identifying ourselves by sex, marital status, financial status, educational level, nationality and even height. We are like video cameras that tape and process what we see around us, yet we are more than just physical beings as we feel and intuit what surrounds us. When sensitivity is a character trait sensory input is interpreted as overload and there is a failure to process these stimuli in a productive way. Instead each event is seen as a possible threat to the system as coping strategies give in to catastrophizing (excessive and exaggerated negative self-statements). As highlighted by Douglas E. DeGood in the *Relationship of Pain-Coping Strategies to Adjustment and Functioning* there have been several studies to show that cognitive-behavioral treatments for chronic pain produce pre-to-post-treatment reduction in catastrophizing.[1] A practice of yoga and meditation with its resultant increase in mindfulness and awareness can be considered a cognitive-behavioral therapy.

According to the *Yoga Sutras of Patanjali*, we are made up of five different *koshas* or levels. Sutras refer to treads, in particular threads of experience that help us develop an understanding of the teachings of yoga. Patanjali was a holy sage credited with being the first to write down these teachings. In the five *koshas* we find our total makeup. Nischala Joy Devi in her book, *The Healing Path of Yoga, Time-Honored Wisdom and Scientifically Proven Methods that Alleviate Stress, Open Your Heart, and Enrich Your Life*, describes these five layers or sheaths in detail.[2] She takes the reader through each sheath in such a way to assist in developing greater relaxation and awareness. By identifying and recognizing these sheaths or levels you can learn to work with the subtle energies of your being and develop internal awareness down to the level of pre-thought impulses or intention. Once you allow yourself to begin playing and experimenting with these energies you can gently release the defensive motives that have you holding on to your pain. Within your center there is no pain. Your job, though your work with yoga and meditation, is to get to your center and function from that place as often as possible.

The first level is the physical level, our body that we are all aware of to varying degrees. We inhabit a physical body that we have to feed, exercise, and rest, to achieve maximum benefit from. The physical body will cry out in pain when it is neglected and will feel energetic after a morning swim at the Y. The physical body will reflect the state of the third body, or the mind body. When we feel sad or depressed we find it difficult to hide these emotions since the body will reflect the inner condition of the mind. Pain etched on the face and in the eyes of the sufferer is evident when we care to look.

The next layer is the energy layer that manifests the life force within us. People with a lot of charisma like Elvis, have active energy levels. This is the layer that gets sapped when we fail to maintain our personal boundaries. It is the layer of *prana* or *chi*, which is the life force. When Obi-wan Kenobi instructed Luke Skywalker to, "Let the force be with you," it was this energy layer that Luke was encouraged to recognize.

Our breath is the representation of *prana* on this plane. With manipulation of the breath we can learn to soften even the tightest, most painful muscles and emotions in our bodies. As mentioned, we hold on to past emotional and physical trauma, but by examining trauma from the perspective of the five different levels we gain greater perspective on the root of such pain. By consciously exhaling the breath through a tense muscle, the movement of the breath sharpens our awareness of how we are holding with muscle contraction. The power of the breath shows us the contribution that we make to our own suffering. Recognizing this, the process of letting go will occur naturally.

One example of how we unconsciously use the breath to hold on occurs when we are taken by surprise or are suddenly frightened. We are at home relaxing, listening to Beethoven's *Moonlight Sonata*, the kids are playing in the adjacent playroom when suddenly a loud thump, followed by a hair-raising scream, shatters the peace of the moment. Knowing there is an eight-foot high loft in the playroom, at the sound of the thump and scream our eyes bulge, muscles tense and instinctively a rapid, sharp, direct in-breath is held. Frozen by the fear, the imagination runs wild. Nothing terrible may have happened and it may just be a scared child, but our system just went into overdrive by reflex. Instead of holding onto the breath let it flow freely to the areas that are calling for healing. Healing will occur naturally if allowed.

The third *kosha* has to do with the mind. It is our minds that we want to learn about. Through understanding its inner workings and natural tendencies the practitioner gains greater insight into individual responsibility, potential, and power. Aware of the root of the incessant chatter we begin to see it for what it is and can choose to stop allowing it to consume our energies. Those who focus on the intellectual aspects of experience do so to avoid painful emotions. In this case it is easier to think things through than it is to deal with conflicting emotions. As these emotions surface they are suppressed and issues are dealt with on a superficial level without feeling.

Like everything else, emotional maturity develops only through practice. To sit quietly in meditation allows you to view your emotions, with all of their varied hues, without the need for responding to them immediately. There is a price to pay for ignoring emotional issues and the price is pain. We limit ourselves by our belief that we are not capable of dealing with these powerful emotions when in fact by intentionally sitting with them and allowing them to surface, through yoga postures, we see they are simply thought without substance.

Part of the healing process involves being able to see this and forgiving ourselves for our own shortcomings. By acknowledging the fact that we did our best under the circumstances we allow ourselves to move on. The mind has many defenses at its disposal, tricking us into doing things the same old way, time after time, even though our current methods are not working for us. Until we see this it is difficult to make any significant progress.

Through daily meditation the ways of the mind are seen. Our circumstances begin to change because of this newfound awareness as we stop doing things and holding on to ideas that have impeded our progress. The mind wants us to do everything we can to avoid suffering and seek out those things that are pleasurable. When we begin to experience greater clarity we see that the mind is what led us into trouble in the first place. From an early age we are told to mind our manners, mind our own business, and mind me or else. Some minds are quicker than others, some are clearer than others, and some are in closer contact with the body than others are. Despite these differences, we can know our own minds through practicing mindfulness.

The fourth level is the wisdom body. This *kosha* is the layer that knows better. We are out of sync when it comes to listening to our own inner wisdom. It is a shame that we are not taught from an early age how to listen to this ever-present knowing. Because we have to slow down and get quiet to listen, it takes too much effort to pay any attention to. So we flounder through life, make more mistakes than we have to, and cause others and ourselves more pain and aggravation than necessary. What we don't know we can learn. There is no need to wait any longer to start listening to this inner voice. It's time to stop telling ourselves that we're too busy, or that we'll wait until vacation, or that there are more important issues to deal with. The sooner we allow our voices to be heard the sooner we find that life and our life experiences are on our side.

Life or God is not the enemy. An untrained mind will exert excess effort and continue going nowhere, spinning its wheels. Lack of mindfulness leads to circular existence, as we are continually confronted with life issues until we have mastered them. The sooner we see this, the sooner we can change direction and move toward inner peace. Let's plant our feet, stand our ground and face our issues. Let them come one at a time, look at them without getting bent out of shape and live.

Meditation will help us find the wisdom that we seek. A poignant Bible passage that can start one on the path to wisdom is, "The fear of the Lord is the beginning of wisdom." We have to wonder what kind of God or Greater Being or Energy would want us to live in fear? A little deeper reading and contemplation leads to the understanding that the word fear means respect.

Respecting the power that we all have is the beginning of wisdom. We each have the power to make our lives wonderful in every way. The converse of this is that we also possess the power to make our lives and the lives of those we love miserable. It is our choice. When we act as if we have forgotten this gem of truth we experience pain and suffering. Sitting quietly with your thoughts and watching your desires, hopes, and fears rise and fall will give you perspective with shinning clarity and acceptance. Once you achieve acceptance a natural unfolding of your nature will take place. As wisdom is allowed to flower you will know what to do and when to do it. You will have a greater awareness of what thoughts, actions, and beliefs allow your pain to continue, worsen, or improve. You will know what lifestyle changes you have to undergo to vibrate on a healthy level. Seek, trust, and believe in your own ability to make things happen and give yourself permission to get this work done through the gifts of yoga and meditation.

The fifth layer is the bliss body. This is the body that we all wish we could continually reside in but act like it doesn't exist. We think it should be handed to us even though we go through our days doing just what we want. We choose not to take time to nourish our minds, we push our bodies to exhaustion and we deny our emotions and treat them like obstacles. The bliss body is always there but it takes practice to enter into this state. Meditation, yoga, prayer, concentration, intention, and restorative time: these are some of the ways to ready ourselves for such a state.

We all move from one layer to the next in random fashion. A good analogy is to liken our energy bodies to the energy levels that electrons occupy in the elements of the periodic table in chemistry. When an electron gains energy it will move up to a higher energy level or orbit. When the electron loses charge is will revert back to a lower level. Awareness of these energy levels helps us to see where our ideas and motivations come from. We are like radio antennas always receiving signals. Until we can fine tune those signals we will come away confused and overwhelmed.

It is easier to begin to understand how and why we view things the way we do when we look at ourselves from more than one level. We are complex, multidimensional beings physically similar in that we have arms, legs, fingers, and toes yet widely different as demonstrated by our unique genetic make-up and individual temperaments and psychological and emotional foundations. There is no one way to understand why we are the way we are. Looking at ourselves as consisting of layers, instead of a solid mass, we can see how a thought or an idea can affect us on different levels. Knowing that the physical body is affected by the condition of the emotional body, and the other four bodies, we can understand why we feel the way we do and why we react the way we do. Just as there are at least two sides to any story there is always more than one reason why we feel the way we do.

In our busyness we forget that we are capable of experiencing a rainbow of emotions. Joy and sadness can be experienced simultaneously. After the death of a loved one, while still in the grieving process, it is possible to continue to feel extreme sadness and great joy. The sense of overwhelming loss and the thought of missed opportunities with our loved ones makes us heavy. Yet as we continue to walk our path awareness grows as we are infused with new life even though our loved one is physically absent. We are richer for having had time to spend with those we love.

Feelings are something that many of us need to get a handle on before we can expect to get to a place where we can feel better about ourselves. The pace of modern day life is not compatible with taking time to sort out the many conflicting feelings we experience. Many times we experience a multitude of feelings simultaneously. These feelings may be ignored simply because it takes too much time and effort, too much introspection to figure them out and sort them out. It would be easier if we had all been trained to automatically process bombarding feelings like a mail sorter might do at the post office. If all of our feelings had zip codes on them we would know where to put them. If our feelings had such codes it would be easier for our brains and neurological machinery to make sense of what is really happening to us. It might take the guesswork and doubt out of much of what we think and do.

It helps to realize that feelings are specific to the individual. No two people will experience the same feeling over a similar event. With different temperaments, expectations, and life experiences we all process events differently. Coming to this realization puts us in a position to learn much from other people. We learn from others because interpretations of shared events may be quite different from ours. We teach others through the same method. Even though none of us will feel the same emotions in response to shared experiences we are all capable of empathy. When your pain is peaking allow yourself to empathize with yourself. Do not choose to continue to ignore your need for recognition. If you don't offer yourself loving kindness first it may be a while before someone else comes along and does it for you. That's a lot of unnecessary suffering.

MEDITATION ON LOVING KINDNESS

Find your quiet place within by focusing on the easy breath. With each exhalation progressively drop all ideas and concepts of who you believe you are. With the settling of the breath begin to ponder who is it that is actually doing the breathing. Let the mind come in concert with the body. Imagine yourself as a newborn baby nestled in the warmth of your mother's arms, embraced and engulfed by her unconditional love. All of your physical, psychological, and emotional needs are met. In this nurturing place you are a perfect being sharing consciousness and bathed in love. Once this vision is achieved and you are comfortable with it take the index finger of your right hand and begin to gently tap the inner aspect of the pinky finger of the right or left hand. Do this just above the base of the fingernail. This point is called the Emergency point and is the distal most portion of the heart meridian.

While you are tapping the H9 point repeat the following affirmation: "I have love and compassion for myself." The heart or fourth chakra is associated with compassion and healing.[3] Through the practice of this exercise you will enable yourself to develop greater compassion and warmth toward yourself and others. This is especially helpful if you constantly get down on yourself or others because you believe that expectations are not being met. With all of the pressures to perform and achieve in today's world, tension and resulting stress are not always

H9 point

expressed appropriately. This leads to unexpressed anger that results in chronic neck pain and headaches. By repeating this procedure you will find that your mind will ease, your expectations will become more realistic and a new friend and ally emerges within your being.

Identifying what our predominant feelings are is possible even if we have lived a life of denial. Learning about feelings is like learning to kayak or fish in that learning is learning. First allow the desire to learn about feelings arise. For men it is not unmanly to develop greater awareness of your feelings. In fact it will help you to be more effective in everything you do especially in relation to work and home life decisions. Your spouse will appreciate the increased sensitivity and your peers will recognize both a strengthening and a softening in your countenance. One might ask why bother about learning more of what my feelings are? In response I would say that to know what you are honestly feeling allows you to be authentic in every encounter you have. It allows you to be honest with yourself. It allows you to live a life of clarity with less confusion and ambiguity. Being in touch with your feelings will keep you from over-extending yourself. It will help you to be impeccable with your word as Dr. Don Miguel Ruiz describes in his book *The Four Agreements*.[iv] This awareness leads to greater self-responsibility without judgement or blame.

When it comes to feelings we can begin to run through a list of specific words that describe best what that feeling is. Our compartment of feeling words is quite limited and small usually consisting of such words as tired, exhausted, crappy, rushed, happy, sad, hungry, and sleepy. When is the last time you used the word elated or for that matter, the word perplexed? Do you recall ever telling someone that you were bedazzled? We seem to have chosen our feeling words sometime ago and closed the book on any attempt at expanding our repertoire. Just because we may be rushed and pressed with the needs of the day we don't have to settle for old worn out words to describe how we feel. The more specific we can be, the more clarity we experience and there is less room for mis-communication.

In the Sanskrit language there are many words that have no English equivalent. The depth of description seems to be greater. As an example, the word *asvasayati* can mean to cause to breathe freely, to comfort, or to console. Another example is the word *cetas*, which can mean mind, heart, intelligence, or understanding. Why not begin to take the time to find deeper meaning in all of the words that you use? We can keep our ears open for new ways to describe the way we feel. In our circle of friends, co-workers, and acquaintances we respond to each other in the same way from day to day. Next time one of these individuals crosses your path make an attempt to relate to them on more than a physical level. See if you can start interpreting their messages on an energetic level and you will walk away with greater understanding. It takes intention and a willingness to try something new and a willingness to be open to new learning, but this new way of perceiving will help you find new ways of problem solving. Expanding your vision opens new vistas and new opportunities as you move into higher energetic levels. Looking at your life and circumstances through a wider-angle lens opens up more possibilities for you now.

When we feel pain, no matter where it is in our bodies, we can use that pain as a source of energy. There may be many times in the course of the day that we check in with our selves and sense exhaustion. Feeling washed out it seems too strenuous just to take another step. At these times when pain makes its presence known, especially in susceptible areas like the cervical neck, periorbital regions, low back, and sternoclidomastoid muscles of the neck, distress levels heighten and it is easy to fall into the habit of catastrophising. Negative thoughts flood your consciousness and the sense that you will never be free of your pain brings you down even lower. Tension on the muscles pulls so hard that it draws the clavicles upward into the neck thus further constricting the cervical spine discs.

Pain is reason enough to have chronic fatigue. There is an incredible amount of energy stored in pain and it can be utilized to get your goals met. It can move you in the direction of being free of your pain. The energy can be used as a teacher to show you how to live and prosper despite any pain you may have had in the past. Redirected energy will transform the perception of the pain from one of dread and agony to hope and excitement. A feeling of renewed confidence moves in and helps replace the sense of helplessness. It is an entirely new way of looking at pain. Pain is energy, but it is frozen energy. In reality we have more energy than we know what to do with but most of it is invested in resisting and fighting off pain. We can all move this energy and put some of it into helping live the life we want to live.

None of this is easy but its better than remaining in the cycle of unrelenting pain. It takes effort and daily concentration to begin to come to a place where you can even begin to look at pain in this way. But what have you got to lose? You have nothing but your pain to lose.

Many times we think that we can wade through a difficult time or situation believing that things will get better later. It is time for us to realize that there may be no later. Now is the only time we have and this may be all that we are going to get. It is time to stop working for another day, to stop living for another day, and start living right now. Start by asking yourself, what do I feel now? I remember as a medical intern in Harrisburg Hospital while on rounds doing SOAP notes. The S was for subjective complaints, O was for objective findings, A was for assessment, and P was for plan. The subjective was the most difficult part to stand through because every little thing that each patient felt I listened to. After some minutes of going through a multitude of ailments it was obvious the patient was not actually feeling all of the terrible symptoms they had elaborately described. As a patient would stop to catch their breath, I would ask, "How do you feel right now?" Since they were looking good when I asked, it was an opportune way to help them contact some of the positive feelings they were having. The fact that they were beginning to feel better had not yet hit home as most of the patients continued to dwell on the symptoms that lead to their admission in the first place. Unknown to me at the time I was trying to assist these individuals in their grounding process. We need to do this for ourselves as much as possible. As we worry about what is to come in an upcoming week, or for that matter the next five minutes, it is easy to get lost living in the future. It comes as a relief to simply check in and ask, "How do I feel now?" Even if you don't feel good at least you have allowed yourself to get in touch with what is real in this moment thus taking yourself out of the state of imagination, fantasy, and delusion.

Dreams are made of the same imagination, fantasy, delusion, illusion, and magic. Everyone dreams but not everyone remembers dreams for a number of reasons. A fear of nightmares, a reflection of overwhelming anxiety, will block dream recall. These blocks can be overcome through the use of auto-suggestion. You can begin to realize that a study of your dreams can be an untapped source of creativity, a reliable problem-solving tool, a forum for rehearsal for important upcoming events, and a source of personal growth.[v]

Most individuals with chronic pain do not sleep soundly. It is believed that in patients with fibromyalgia, disordered sleep patterns are a contributing factor to the progression of symptoms as the lack of restful sleep leads to greater fatigue and a lower pain tolerance. Fibromyalgia patients tend to have reduced REM (rapid eye movement) sleep and as well as disturbances in non-REM or restorative sleep (Stage IV sleep). Stage IV sleep is were we have our deepest sleep. It is hard to awaken from this stage of sleep. It is the sleep you experience when you are awakened by a middle of the night phone call and you are groggy, finding it hard to listen to what is being said and hard to put your thoughts together. This stage of sleep is associated with delta waves on an electroencephalogram (EEG). In fibromyalgia, stage III and IV sleep has more alpha activity (the brain wave pattern seen in light sleep) than it should thus there is less restful sleep.

Dreaming occurs during REM sleep. In the *Yoga Sutras of Pantanjali* it is described as one of the five activities of the mind. The other four activities being comprehension, misapprehension, imagination, and memory. Sleep is like everything in life. It is like the four seasons that in one night we go from one stage of sleep to the next. Any disruption in one stage will lead to disruption in the successive stages. On an EEG in non-REM or slow-wave sleep we find four stages. Sleep deepens from stage I to IV with progressively slower brain wave activity. Once REM sleep is achieved, usually ninety minutes after going to sleep, the activity of the brain is markedly increased. This lasts for five to ten minutes. Most adults have five to six sleep cycles per night with each cycle having longer REM periods than the previous cycle.

Why not use these nighttime hours to assist in self-healing. We spend one third of our life asleep. The major hurtle to overcome is getting over the fear of what you might discover. This is where meditation and the yoga poses will help in that daily practice will demonstrate that it is not harmful to stay with whatever emotions or feelings arise. With practice you are able to foster the attitude of being a warrior. You reconnect with the true source of power within that is always present and available to you, but that in the past with all of the preoccupation with stress and worry you have forgotten about.

In order to develop increased awareness of our sleep states it is necessary to begin with the intention. When it is time to retire at night a few common sense steps will lead you into the mindset of restful sleep. First do not try to go to sleep with the television on or with music playing. It is fine to listen to soothing music of your choice just prior to sleep but once you settle in and are ready for sleep turn off the radio or CD player. Also turn off all of the lights unless you are an advanced practitioner of dream yoga when a small light on allows for increased awareness. Avoid caffeinated products for at least three to four hours prior to sleep. Do your best to avoid reading anything that might be stimulating to the imagination such as mystery novels. Do not try to tackle any difficult reading that would have the effect of over engaging your mind.

Prepare to write down your dreams by having a pen and pad at the bedside. If you think you are going to get up and find a paper and pen in the middle of the night you are only fooling yourself. Have these tools ready and if possible have a small book reading light so that you do not have to turn on bright lamps or lights. At times writing down a single word is enough to help stimulate your mind to recall the bulk of your dream thus allowing you to wait until the morning to recount the entire dream sequence.

Every part of your dream is a part of you. This is true even when there is someone else in your dream field. The intimate and hidden messages that are yours and yours alone are to be found in your sleeping hours. You do not need a book of dream interpretations to tell you what your dreams mean. If you are willing to fearlessly look at the content of your dreams with honesty in the context of your situation, needs, wants, and desires, you will know what your dreams are trying to tell you. View them as a wise counselor or helper who will always be there.

Most people feel powerless over their dreams thinking that bad dreams or recurring troublesome dreams come to them for unknown reasons. The reality is that you have total control over what you dream if you just exercise that practice. When reading the Buddhist texts we gain exposure to the idea that we are dreaming most if not all of the time. As we go through our day we find that our waking thoughts are no different than the stuff that our dreams are made of. Unless we practice mindfulness and choose to remain present in each moment, our waking hours are just as dream-like as the contents of our dreams.

Tenzin Wangyal Rinpoche tells us in *The Tibetan Yogas of Dream and Sleep*, there is nothing more real than dream.[vi] If we move through life and never question our individual and cultural beliefs then we dull consciousness and continue living the dream. Cultivation of awareness and recognition of the dualistic nature of our thinking brings us out of the dream. We all want more pleasure and less pain. We label one thing good and the other bad thus missing out on the direct experience that life has to offer. Can you now generate a new braveness and see what is truly in front of you without labels? Have you taken the time and made the effort to figure out whose dream you have been living? Ask this of yourself as you prepare to dream tonight.

You have the power to undo any and all negative impressions, aversions, ill feeling, and discontent that you have ingrained in your make up. This is achieved by recreating positive conditions in your mind during your dream periods. When you find yourself falling in a dream, once you are aware that you are in control, you can change that sensation of falling into the feeling of flight. In order to release any negative impressions you have to be willing to let go of grasping. This means you let go of grasping for more of anything that you deem pleasurable. You have to also release the impressions of aversion. You have to be willing to empty yourself and get comfortable with the feeling of emptiness, which paradoxically leaves you feeling fulfilled and complete. There is a place of neutrality that can be maintained, at first with great effort, but then with increasing spontaneity. The time that you spend in meditation and the intentional relaxation of all effort in your yoga practice will show you how to move forward with increasing compassion.

Developing compassion for yourself will have you choosing to fly in your dream instead of falling. Compassion for an angry spouse, boss, coworker, or customer will have you understanding their fear as well as yours. To awaken compassion it takes a new way of thinking. It is necessary to drop old belief systems that tell you it is mandatory to be tough to survive. You have to be willing to lighten up. For those with pain the suggestion to lighten up is the last thing they want to hear, thinking how can I lighten up when I have so much terrible pain? It is necessary to trust the process. Pain develops because muscles are tense. They get balled and knotted up when they are not given a chance to relax, release, and let go. Their blood supply gets cut off and they ache. Their sensory nerve innervation becomes over stimulated to the point of numbness. The mind gets caught up in the pain cycle and it believes that you will never get rid of the pain. In the dream you take the mind out of play and let your soul, your being, do the healing. You know what you need. Allow it to happen.

Each night before bed tell yourself gently that you will remain open and aware of what your dreams need to tell you about yourself. The grounding that you have gained from the discipline of daily yoga and meditation will allow you to stand your ground in the face of the fear that will arise. Standing firm as the warrior, fear will fall away and you will be free.

It helps to immerse yourself in reading texts that are meant to generate compassion. This concept was understood by our third president Thomas Jefferson when he wrote, "I never go to bed without an hour, or half hour's, previous reading of something moral."[vii] Books that teach you to meditate can be found everywhere these days. The Internet is loaded with web sites that explain the different styles of meditation. Choose one style and see if it fits. If not, move to another school of meditation until you find the one that is right for you. Don't worry if you do not have a teacher at first. Allow this book to be your first teacher and tutor. With continued focus and interest you will be led to the next step that may possibly be a magazine article, then a formal yoga or meditation class and possibly a weekend retreat. Pema Chodron, an American Buddhist nun and prolific author on the subject of meditation and the development of compassion tells us that we have to, "Start Where You Are."[viii] Things will unfold as you sow these seeds of emotional release. You will find yourself more present and mindful as you continue to practice. It is only when you acknowledge just how scared you are or just how much pain you are experiencing that you open the door to change. Explore all avenues, leave no stone unturned when it comes to increasing you awareness. These steps will free you and even allow you to live joyfully with your pain.

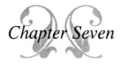

Chapter Seven

In the Now: Surrender

*S*o here you are in the now. What do you do right now that you find yourself here? Wait a minute and you're no longer in the now. It is so easy to move away from the present moment. Fantastic battles are conjured up in our heads worrying about what will be expected of us tomorrow. We do not like being in the now. It's too scary, maybe too real for us to feel safe. What is considered safe is based on past experiences making very little room for anything new. It is a shame that we feel safer living with old ideas, which in reality are dead and gone, or in the future that may never come.

Fear of the present is related to an inability to deal with feelings and needs. At times anger keeps us from being present. At other times it is an inability to stand up to others for what we think instead of folding to their wants. In such a place remaining in the present in not possible because of the ongoing internal argument, an argument we can not win. We fight and fight. We talk back and forth to an unseen energy and deplete ourselves ending up drained. We're left wondering why we are so tired. At the end of the day, even with a day off from work, there is only exhaustion. It is the internal battle that is wearing us out.

Sometimes we feel we may never win. We think we want to be in the moment, but the second we realize that we are finally in this moment we blow it for ourselves and revert back to old learned ways of making trouble for ourselves. It is as if we like and thrive on turbulence. If we can't see the hurricane coming, by God, we'll generate one. Our minds race in internal argument like a category V hurricane, blowing all sensibility out of reach. It is as if we are not happy unless there is constant drama in our lives. Maybe we think we are not fully alive if our lives are not going along like a soap opera. People get bored in their marriages. Each partner goes off on his or her own tangent, with his or her own interests, and before you know it you're making up scenarios as to why your partner's life is so much better than yours. You begin to stop listening to each other and when you do speak you think you know what your partner is going to say before they say it. You have lost the ability to listen. The same thing happens when you get into the now and you don't listen to what is going on inside right at that moment. You block out the moment by jumping to another time. Who needs a time machine to get away from the real issues when we have our own imaginations?

To stay in the moment the first criteria required is to want to be in the moment. There are energies within each of us that we do not understand. When we begin to acknowledge our ignorance we begin to see what is really going on. Here I am again. What should I do? Should I bask in the bliss of the moment and just hang out and see what happens? Or should I bail out and jump to another time because I can't take what is happening now? Moments follow moments and no two are ever the same, but we are so good at making generalizations that each moment seems just like the one past so nothing ever seems new to us. Is that why we seek out more exciting movies, more exciting sports, more exciting partners, and more exciting lives?

As I was growing up kids were just beginning to use skateboards. Now there are pros like Tony Hawk who can skateboard better than most people can walk. In order for him to perfect his technique he had to continuously return to the moment. To get his program right he had to seek out the rough spots and make the necessary corrections. He puts on a good show because he knows how to stay focused and in the moment. Remaining present is a full time job, but there is no reason why it has to be hard work. It only seems that way now because we are not used to thinking in this manner. The more we appreciate all of the beauty that surrounds us the easier it is to stay

114

conscious. The more we intently focus on the task at hand, the more present we will be.

Just because an event occurring in the present is viewed as negative, or unfortunate, it might in the long run turn out to be beneficial. A good example of this is when someone loses his or her job. Initially it is felt that is a huge inconvenience as there is a family to support, a mortgage to pay, and all the other bills to cover that won't just go away. This new condition, though stressful, can be used as an opportunity to move into a new area of interest. Such unexpected events can be viewed as new opportunities that will lead to new awakenings and new avenues of questioning that would not have surfaced if the event had not occurred.

Time can be spent getting to know your spouse and family better. It is a time to make more space for yourself and allow your passions to brew. What passion is your pain trying to reignite in you? It is an especially good time to regenerate if you had been forcing yourself to go to a job that took more away from you than you could safely give. Such situations only lead to greater pain leaving you with a suppressed immune system and more prone to illness.

Those individuals working in a state of chronic pain find it difficult to get things done as efficiently as they would like. Much of their time is spent in necessary self-talk to keep the pain manageable. If built in breaks are not allowed the pain only intensifies with the result being increasing frustration. This emotion is not easily forgotten or shed since the pain memory is so ingrained. What is needed is rest and recuperation. Time alone in silence is the best way to drop down the level of the pain. Attention to the breath will lead you back into the now and help you manage your discomfort.

For various reasons we find we are not comfortable in the moment. The closer to the moment we get it seems that our anxiety becomes more acute. It's like a pilot approaching the eye of a hurricane. The most turbulent and powerful winds are around the eye but once into the eye there is complete calm. The anxiety may not be getting more acute but we become more aware of the totality of it. When we approach the moment things may not be to our liking. When this happens it is all the more reason to get out of the moment and move the mind to a place that is more pleasing. You don't like what someone is saying because it hooks something from the past so they're tuned out. They stop talking to you and later you find they don't care to speak with you at all. You hurt and can't seem to figure out why.

IN THE MOMENT MEDITATION AND ASANA

This asana and meditation can be performed anytime to help you bring yourself back into the present moment. Begin by finding a quiet place where you can be undisturbed for at least five minutes. If possible remove your shoes to allow unimpeded contact with the floor or ground. With your toes pointing straight ahead, place your feet shoulder width apart. Take a deep inhalation in through your nose. As you begin the exhalation allow your torso to flow forward. If possible allow your palms to gently touch the floor. If this deep a forward bend (Uttanasana) is not achievable at this time, place the palms on the shins as close to the ankles as they will reach without straining. If reaching for the shins is too much of a stretch then rest your palms on your thighs.

With the forward bend you will feel pressure in the lower abdominal region, back of the thighs, lower back, and neck. Use the movement of your breath on the exhalation to release this pressure thus allowing the muscles to lengthen. Feel your feet anchored to the floor as you allow the weight of your head to deepen the bend. As you take long and slow in breaths feel the pressure build to a crescendo. At the end of the in breath ask yourself where you are holding on at this moment. Observe the dialogue between the body and mind, and then allow the pressure to once again dissipate on a slow intentional exhalation.

Receive another slow, quite, and unforced in breath and ask yourself what you have to do to bring comfort to the areas of unwanted pressure. Do not try to force yourself to relieve any discomfort but instead observe and listen to your inner wisdom. It may simply be an idea that you will be directed to let go of that will bring you balance. What expectations are you holding yourself to that may be keeping you from being ever-present? Are there expectations of others that are at the root of your absence?

Just observe, pay attention and see and feel for yourself what is going on for you right now.

The forward bend is a relaxing and calming asana. As you question yourself, look upon your internal television screen to see what images arise. In this posture you can remain with whatever impressions come up. See the vision then slowly open your eyes and look at your hands, your feet, and the floor. Sense your surroundings, listen for any extraneous noise, and then check in with your body again for any pain or discomfort. In the presence of that pain know that you are currently one with it. Do not try to make it go away but accept that it is present and that it wants to assist you in being evermore present. Close your eyes gently once again and exhale through your pain or discomfort. Maintain slow, easy exhalations, keeping your mind and body soft, yet supported by the definite contact with the ground. Think ease. Feel ease. Be ease. When you are ready, open your eyes, stand up slowly and maintain the sense of ease as you continue on with your day.

There are too many feelings going on within each of us at any one time to pay attention to all of them. In modern day life with all that we are occupied with during the course of our day we attend to only the predominant emotions and feelings at any one time. Knowing that there are many facets to what we are feeling allows us to look at our feelings as if they were the colors of the spectrum or a painter's pallet. As the painter continues to paint, the colors on the pallet begin to intermix and blend into each other. The brush goes from color to color as the painter continually fine tunes what he wants to see on the canvas. The artist knows that blue is not just blue, and red is not just red. Aware of the different hues, mixing a little white with blue brings a softer blue, a blue seen in the midmorning sky over the ocean on a Sunday. He knows just how to produce a powder blue that is just short of white and that only looks blue because of the contrast from the surrounding white of the clouds. Whenever we look at the sky it is always the only time it will ever look just that way. In it there are many shades of blue, a touch of purple here and there; some smaller patches of gray and pure white where the sun has melted through the otherwise cloud covered sky. The layers of clouds look like the skin of a snake at one moment then in the next moment they resemble the outline of the Himalayas from a great distance.

So it is with our feelings and our thoughts. They are constantly changing and never just composed of one thing, as solid as a rock, but are a blend of all that we have known before and all that we hope to know. All past experiences, all past thoughts, all   expectations and hopes dance together in a rhythm created by our own vibrations to make us who we are. This process is not static, but is made static and solid when we hold on to painful memories, sensations, and thoughts. Nothing about being human has to be solid. If we think in that way then we have made it solid and rigid. Firm and hard in our old ways we limit our possibilities for the future. We limit our capacity for enjoyment. We limit what can come to us and what we can comprehend. We effectively close off our consciousness.

Right now is there anything you can tell yourself that would make your world perfect? Right now can you accept your circumstances and be thankful for what has been given to you? You may have made a mess of things in the past, but the place to start your reconstruction project is in the now. Think about what you are. You are one of the most sophisticated beings on this planet with a mind, a body, and a soul whose purpose is to fulfill your purpose. You are you and that is enough. Now is the time to realize this as our time is fleeting and limited. It is your choice to live in the moment or to waste your time in the past trying to relive things the way you think they should have been. It does nothing for your effectiveness to live in the future either. It is good to plan for the future but the only way to make changes for the future is to do it in the now.

What are you waiting for? The perfect moment is now. Many folks avoid productive endeavors by using the excuse that the weather is no good. If it's too hot then that is a good enough excuse to stay in and watch TV. If it's too cold, it's not worth the risk of getting out there and catching a cold. It is beneficial to work in the yard, or go for walks in nature as it helps us ground. We are more likely to be reminded of our place in the world by direct contact with the outside. It helps us get out of our heads and into our hearts. You don't have to be a professional to start your intended project. Get out there, dig up the dirt, sift it, and plant some seeds. The seeds to your healthier, happier, more fulfilling life are within you now.

Drop your need to be a perfectionist and support your intention to stay with a project. Drop what ever excuses that are keeping you from starting a meditation and yoga program. Excuses are simply reasons not to act. Momentarily surrender your excuses and watch what thoughts and feeling come to you. Then take action. Don't wait for the perfect day because every-day is a perfect day. Get into the habit of labeling all of your circumstances as perfect for you. Even your pain right now is perfect as it has a message. Open to it and make space within for the transformation that will naturally follow.

During hurricane Isabel, my then three year old, Joel, wanted to go out-side and play in the wind. He saw the trees swaying, he saw the leaves zip-ping by at seventy miles an hour and he thought it would be a good day to go out and experiment with the wind. We all need to keep that child within alive. Not that I allowed Joel to go out and play but I did appreciate his desire to learn more about the world in which he lives. It is time to appreci-ate your curiosity and capacity to learn. To conquer your pain you have to be willing to get over your fear of it and learn about it. It is already your com-panion. Why not make it a friendly companion?

The way to most help yourself is to come into the now and ask yourself what it is you need right now. If you need to be left alone, for whatever rea-son, then tell those around you that you need some time for yourself. Even if you can only get away for five minutes, those five minutes may be the best five minutes of your day. The insights gained can make the rest of your day more enjoyable. The lives of those around you will improve in the process. If you find yourself mulling over events of the past, acknowledge that fact and listen to yourself. Your inner being knows what you need. The multiple aspects of your being are doing what they think they need to keep you func-tioning. Unfortunately many times those parts are not working together. They may have the same goal, survival of the self, but their means may be very different. Their likes and dislikes are also very different. It is like the FBI and the CIA when it comes to tracking terrorist activity. If the left hand doesn't know what the right hand is doing then they may be doing twice the work. One organization may have one piece of the puzzle, which alone makes no sense, but put the two pieces together and a solution may be more apparent. So it is with each of us. Parts of us may know what to do but if the other parts keep that part down then there is chronic frustration. The frustration leads to anger and the anger leads to alienation, loneliness, and persistent pain.

Now is the time to start living. Now is the time to look at what you want to do and take the steps to get things moving in that direction. It doesn't make any difference what your past was like; in fact you can use what you have learned to help you trek ahead. The mistakes you think you made in the past were actually your teachers. You can thank yourself for allowing those mistakes, knowing that you don't have to make them again. Now is the time to move. Now is the time to sit and meditate. Look at and listen to what comes up. There will be a multitude of thoughts, feelings, and inner pictures, past fears, joys, doubts, and successes. Listen and stay open. Choose to pay attention to even the quietest nudging. Do not disregard anything that comes up, good or bad. Even if you think, that can't be, look deeper and see where it takes you.

Have no limits for you are a creator. Go wherever it is that you need to go. When fear arises, look at that also. Where has the fear come from? What is the source of the fear? You will find that the fear comes from within. We choose what we will be afraid of. Since we are the one's who choose what to fear it goes to follow that we are the one's to chose what not to be afraid of. When we are unable to see this then fear persists and it keeps us from living fuller lives. Stuck and crying for help, we continue to feel pain. It is time to wake up and realize that we are the only one's capable of helping ourselves. We can call on others to assist but in the final analysis we are the ones who will make the final decision.

On a white water rafting trip we floated north down the French Broad River. We stopped downstream and those who wanted were able to climb a large rock and jump off into the river. In the past I would have never entertained the thought of jumping off such a rock. That kind of thing was for someone else. Why risk my body by jumping off a rock? Now with my desire to grow and to find new ways and things to experience the chance to jump off a rock was viewed as an opportunity to experience something new. The choices were to sit in the raft and watch everyone else having fun, or get out of the boat, face the expected fears and learn something. By choosing to act you find that others share similar fears.

There are healthy fears, fears grounded in reality. You better be afraid if you are a firefighter about to run into a burning building because you know someone is still inside. That fear will help sharpen your senses and guide you toward making the right decisions, which may keep you alive. Such fear will give your body more strength and energy than you would otherwise be able to muster without the fear. In this case you have a better chance of getting your goal accomplished through the energy within the fear. Other times ungrounded fear may keep you from ever acting. You will sit with your fear wondering what might have been if you didn't feel the fear and if you had only had the guts to act despite it. The more you fight your fear and pain the stronger they get.

There are not many of us that know the meaning of the word surrender. Infrequently used in the American vocabulary, it is not a word we keep in our consciousness. When I hear "surrender," I think of the Japanese signing the terms of surrender on the battleship Missouri at the end of World War II after Harry Truman decided to drop the Little Boy and the Fat Boy atomic bombs on Hiroshima and Nagasaki. The word is not compatible with American life. We are driven to do well in school from the beginning. Today parents are priming their children for college entrance exams while they are still in grammar school. Parents and grandparents want their offspring attending the most prestigious colleges thinking such institutions will ensure success. Nothing succeeds like a degree from the Wharton School of Business or from Harvard.

In sports all team members are taught to fight until the end and not give up even though they are losing by an insurmountable number of points. Encouraged to continue fighting, cancer patients are geared by society to never surrender to their disease. New anti-cancer agents, forever being developed, are expected to be the best and the newest in the armamentarium against cancer.

What is wrong with the idea of surrendering? Are we too afraid to let what is going to naturally happen just happen? Maybe we all feel that we need to exert as much control over our lives as possible as we cannot trust a higher power to take care of us the way we expect to be taken care of. To surrender is to stop fighting. So much wasted effort and so much worry could be avoided if we all just surrender to what is. Otherwise we end up fighting ourselves. It takes trust to allow what is to be. Maybe we don't trust ourselves or maybe we don't trust God or the universe.

To surrender is not to give up or lose all hope. It is to let be what is going to be, accepting what is happening right now for what it is, without judgement or desire for something else. It is allowing ourselves to be where we are and not wishing that we were somewhere else or somebody else. Surrender is a tall order, not something we are taught, but something we can continually work toward.

What better time to practice surrender than during meditation. I say practice because this is all we can do. As we get comfortable with the idea of surrender we carry the concept into our daily routine and begin to allow what is happening to unfold the way it is going to unfold without undue angst about it. During meditation, sitting with the breath and being still, as a thought or idea comes up we can tell ourselves to give into the current thought. We do not try to resist or change the thought. We do not to tell ourselves that the thought is good or bad but just observe the thought, follow it and let it proceed to its end. Do not fear letting go of it as another thought will arise. This is what a normal functioning mind does. We suffer when we try to hold on to thoughts and ideas or concepts. When we can get big enough and develop enough confidence in what we are doing in our meditation then we allow surrender to take place. Until we make a decision to release our struggle we will continue to fight and resist what is. Such behavior is a waste of energy. It makes us tired and cranky.

To surrender is to give up our preconceived needs. It is not to stop taking care of ourselves. It is to realize what our real needs are like feeling part of a family, part of a community, part of the human race and going about our day with concern about how our actions and our beliefs effect everyone else. Surrendering is telling ourselves that this moment is enough, that we are complete without anything extra. Even though we may not have the whitest teeth or the newest fashions, or the car of the year, what we are at this moment is enough. When we realize and believe this then we rid ourselves of the duality of life. We can say I AM. We can say I AM without any classifier tagged on to build us up bigger than we really are because we are already big enough.

To surrender is to say I am good enough. No one has to settle for mediocrity knowing that each one of us is perfect for what we are. When we can relax with this thought things are allowed to naturally fall into place and come our way without the added effort that we think we need to contribute. Everything takes effort but I am talking about effortless effort. During a yoga retreat in California I was one of three people in the class who were not yoga teachers. I had spent most of the prior year doing restorative yoga because of the nature and long hours required of my work. This was the first seven-day yoga retreat that I had ever participated in so I knew that I would need a special mindset to help me through the process. A few days before leaving for the retreat I was reading through the Sutras of Pantanjali and came across the verse concerning the asanas or postures. The idea that I decided to focus on while working on the asanas was to, "Relax all effort and keep the minds attention on the infinite." This one phrase helped me to surrender to each moment as it came up during our long practice sessions. It helped me to relax into the poses and not have one muscle group fight another muscle group, which would have caused undue fatigue. Surrendering to the moment freed me from thinking how hard I thought I had to work to achieve a posture. Instead of working to get into the pose I allowed the phrase and the breath to lead me from one moment to the next, like a movie film would move from frame to frame with no one point static.

We are always in motion even when we think we are holding a pose. In holding a pose if we allow ourselves to surrender to our vibrations we can clearly feel that we are not static. That vibration is life happening. That movement is life happening. Surrendering to these moments we feel alive. The trick is to carry these ideas and states of being into our daily lives. As we are able to do this our experience of life blossoms.

In surrendering to the moment we give up the notion that we have to project ourselves into an illusionary future. We can ask ourselves, where are we now? We can be satisfied with our answer: we are right here. This is what Jon Kabat-Zinn was referring to in his popular book titled *Wherever*

You Go, There You Are. Surrender is about mindfulness and being present. Many people stare into space a lot as if in a trance. It is admirable to ponder on noble thoughts, but when the staring is used as a means of escaping from the present moment it acts as a thief robbing you of your precious experience of life. We have all heard about the good old days from well-meaning relatives and friends and maybe that is what some people need to cope with their issues. For myself, I find that I am more effective to myself and those around me the more I can stay in the moment. Being present you help yourself and those you are dealing with. This is especially so in a medical oncology practice setting where individuals are dealing with quality of life issues on a moment to moment basis.

Grasping onto the past or projecting ourselves into the future is so far removed from surrendering to the moment. It is more like giving up on the moment. We are all bigger than that but need to be willing to see that. By surrendering our old ideas about what life is all about and by surrendering our stories we begin to experience what it is to be present. We can decide to drop in on this moment. If it happens to be scary for whatever reason we can look at it calmly and take the steps to stay with the fear. It is wiser to hold our ground and face the fears that come up for then we see that our fears are just a projection of the mind. We begin to see that we are not our fears.

Surrendering to who we are is an active process. It will not come naturally. We have to work at it. Just like anything else the more we practice, the better we get. In the beginning there will be periods of frustration and the frustration will rise again and again. Even when we think we are beginning to get good at it there will be some backsliding as there is in everything. As we get better at surrendering to the moment we find our energy levels rise. We see the direction we are meant to go and events unfold with less worry and debate. Our own voice will be more audible as the infighting and inner conflict begins to resolve and abate. The clock is ticking and it is time to begin the work of surrender.

Choose to begin to see some of the inner defenses for what they are; barriers to who you really are and what you really need and want. Consciously relaxing the base of the tongue will quite the chatter that keeps your energies dispersed and keeps you from being as effective as possible.

Surrender to the quiet within and feel the expansion of consciousness begin to flood your being as the total experiences of your life come together to make you whole. We remember everything that has ever happened to us. In making this greater awareness the ultimate goal and as we surrender our ignorance we can move toward greater acceptance of ourselves. It is never too late to surrender and give up the inner fight, the inner battle that we have been fighting all in an effort to prove our reason for being. There is no need to prove anything.

Surrender and see what is really going on. Our role in our drama is the lead role. It is the only part we can change, but before we can change we need to see exactly what we are doing to ourselves. Surrendering drops all pretenses. Surrender is a decision not to judge or criticize. Surrender has the power of thunder immediately able to crack our toughest parts and soften them into acceptance. We can surrender now and drop all ideas of who we are. Then we are free to experience our true essence and our oneness with everything becomes obvious. In such a place there is no holding on to anger, fear, frustration, jealousy or any other harmful emotion. In such a place the sound of the universe is heard above all other sounds and that sound is within all of us. Allowing our own vibrations to happen, we dissolve into the infinite and realize this very moment is the good old days.

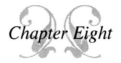

Chapter Eight

Effort

*W*hen everything we do and all our efforts never seem to make a difference, it is easy to think: what's the use? In taking steps to bring about positive change one can expect times of set back and overwhelming depression. When nothing we say or think seems to make a difference then all of our energy has to be shifted to finding ways to feel better. This does not mean that we deny what we are feeling. Instead bringing the feeling in line with reality allows dissipation of the disparity between the two. The expenditure of effort is toward dropping expectations, not in some action to be taken.

During these stressful moments, what change in attitude can you embrace to feel better about your situation? The demands of the day already find you taxed and there is no extra effort left that you can make. You keep going putting one foot in front of the other. Momentarily getting a brief respite, later to find the heavy burdens persist and never really go away. The constant struggle to discover an underlying reason for all of this pain and suffering keeps you wondering just what life is all about. Many times it is the little things that tee us off, like being handed unexpected work or not getting an anticipated day off. Constant fatigue makes the little things seems much bigger than they are, but no matter how minor the irritation, the same frustration and anger rips up any thoughts of contentment.

Contentment can be measured in degrees and even the smallest degree can give reason for hope. Living without contentment leads to chronic depression, anxiety, and recurring pain. Confused over how or where to apply your effort, you are left with the belief that you are powerless to change anything. It is like being lost in a foreign city without a road map or being driven for miles and miles making twists and turns on unfamiliar roads only to be dropped off on a deserted dirt road on a moonless night. Like a blind person in the middle of Times Square, one step in the wrong direction and it's all over. In the dark, feeling your way without a destination, bumping into obstacles and getting hurt, you are lost. Wandering without a charted course there is no purpose in what you are doing. Without focus and intention there is no concerted effort or direction of thought so you are left to lick your wounds and suffer for reasons you know not why.

There are many theories as to why we developed as a human race but nobody knows why for sure and we probably will never know. Such is the uncertainty which we have to exist living hour to hour, day to day, week to week, month to month, and year to year. The only things we can be sure of are that as we get older time passes more quickly and we are all going to die. No matter how hard some of us try to deny this fact, no one is will be exempt and find themselves living forever. What happens next is anyone's guess.

Why bother putting out effort doing something that does not feed you if in the end it won't make any difference? Why not put your energies into the things that please you and fill you? It comes back to the idea of being in the now because that is the only certainty that any of us have. There is no promise that the next breath is coming, so make the choice to savor this breath as if it were your last.

In the same vein, Steven Levin explains in *One Year to Live*, we need to make the best of what we are given. What's the use in worrying about tomorrow if it may never come? There is nothing to gain by excessive self-sacrifice to the point that we deny ourselves enjoyment and satisfaction today. We should not live in total disregard for tomorrow but if our goal is always to prepare for tomorrow at the expense of living fully today, then we are on the wrong track. We are on a track to disillusionment and despair.

Life is not compatible with coasting for the long term. There may be times, after great effort, when achievements are made and we can take it easy for a while, but we find that more will be asked of us at a later date.

Our minds are always going, moving to the next idea. In our meditation practice and in the activities that we choose during our days, there is no point in trying to totally calm the mind because that will never happen. We can watch the mind, notice the calmness around the mind and decide to drop the mind into that calm.

In making an effort to quiet the mind, this effort in itself is taken by the mind as a signal to activate and get prepared. It makes the mind more noisy. Let the mind do what it wants, yet observe it without getting wrapped up in its story. Peace and contentment will come from staying centered. There is no benefit in fighting our natures. The mind can be tamed only to a degree. The rest of the time we have to put out effort to keep it focused and concentrated. This comes with practice, patience, and gentleness. The Buddha put all of his efforts into training his mind in such a way.

In order to go about your business with optimal effort, in ways that will bring you maximum joy and minimal pain, it is necessary to be aware of your contribution to your condition. The Buddha spoke about Right View and Right Effort. On the path to freedom you are given directions. These road signs are found in the discourse of the Noble Eightfold Path. The path he describes is actually the practice of a set of attitudes that will lead to liberation from suffering. The Noble Eightfold Path encompasses the following: Right View, Right Thinking, Right Speech, Right Action, Right Livelihood, Right Effort, Right Mindfulness, and Right Concentration. When these factors are practiced then "joy, peace, and insight will be there."[2]

If something is not working in your life, a certain mind set or belief is allowing continued pain and suffering. It is possible to drop this way of thinking and replace it with Right View. Right View is the first of the eight path factors in the Noble Eightfold Path. It belongs to the wisdom division of the path and concerns itself with knowledge regarding stress. In order to remove undue stress from your life it is important to realize what you think or do in your waking moments that lead to the generation of stress. It is necessary to be aware of what thoughts and actions are conducive to the cessation of stress. To live with Right View a practitioner has to continually contemplate the ways leading to the cessation of stress.

Pain is a stimulus. If you allow yourself to view your pain as something to get over instead of something that has a message for you; that is wrong view. Pain comes into your life insidiously, but once rooted in your psyche, it will make your life miserable. By momentarily putting your fear aside and patiently listening, your pain will show you where to place your effort and attention. Pain speaks to you by informing you about what you have to let go of. It will speak to you of suffering as long as you continue to resist it.

In quieting the mind you are able to see the defensive postures you have been taking in an attempt to keep pain at bay. This is possible because once you are able to view your fear as thought substance, and not as reality, you gain the courage to look deeply at your pain. When you look at your pain and feel it, with even greater intensity, do not let that stop you from looking even deeper. You will find clarity, peace, and passion when you face your pain with consistency and Right View.

You bring persistent pain and struggle into your life when you dwell on the issues of "I" and the self. When you question your past, question your future, and continually ponder who you are then you are bound to the wheel of life and rebirth or samsasra. These thoughts lead to doubt and grasping which are both conducive to pain and suffering.

The same idea follows when you are having pain and continually question why it is that you are having this pain. It is good to initially ask why this pain has come upon you, but to persistently ask this only leads to more pain. A wiser path to follow is to ask what you can do to stop your pain. First recognize that your pain is stress. Ask what beliefs or thoughts have led to the stress. Then inquire as to what it will take to remove the stress in the form of what ideas or beliefs you can drop. This will help to melt away the stress. Continue practicing by generating and holding views that lead to non-confusion, increase, plenitude, and joy.

To live with chronic physical pain is to suffer. The pain associated with depression, anxiety, disappointment, and frustration results in the same sense of suffering. In the Four Noble Truths, the Buddha taught that life is insepa-rably linked to suffering or *dukkha*. This term encompasses all kinds and degrees of suffering including the feeling that life is just not what you thought it should be. As you get older the idealistic thoughts concerning your role in the world seem to dim and a growing sense of dissatisfaction expands. Through the continual practice of The Eightfold Path it is possible to supplant your dissatisfaction with a passion for life as you experience greater degrees of liberation from suffering.

No one wants to consciously suffer but there are forces and motivations well below the level of awareness that will only make themselves know to you through conscious work and effort. The seed to begin this exploration has to be planted and tended by you and only you. Along the way help is available through counselors, family members, relatives, friends and teachers of meditation and yoga, as well as books, articles, videos, CD's and tapes.

To say that you want peace in your life with one breath then to turn around and tell someone that your task at hand is a pain in the neck is not consistent with Right View or Right Speech. Intention has to match thought, word, and action for you to experience joy and freedom from suffering. Habits are so deeply ingrained over time that their sometime harmful natures are not seen by the untrained mind. Looking at the narrow road ahead, from where you are to where you want to go, may be overwhelming, but by making an effort to examine your own ignorance the path will widen.

With our preoccupation with doing, I have chosen to discuss in some detail the concept of Right Effort next. It is the fifth factor in the Eightfold Path which helps us to cultivate wisdom and dissolve ignorance. In taking the first steps to overcome pain the path will reveal itself more clearly if you realize that the goal is the end of suffering through the cultivation of wisdom. Your pain will ease its grip on you in proportion to the degree of wisdom that you develop through your practice. To make room for wisdom it is necessary to recognize just how engulfed the mind is with greed, aversion, and delusion. Such delicate examination is possible only through consciously quieting the mind through daily meditation.

Effort is energy. In chapter three we discussed ways of finding new sources of energy through working with the *chakra* system. By recognizing the potential energy stores within through concentrated effort these sources of strength, clarity, and direction can be tapped leading to greater fulfillment. In making the effort to practice acceptance of current beliefs, the door is opened wider to positive change. For most folks acceptance does not come easy as it takes repetitive, directed effort to move in this direction. Here we will find ways to direct this energy and put our effort to work in a balanced way.

In the daily attempts at dropping the desires of ego, the persistence of pleasure and the aversion of pain, one of the most difficult aspects to let go of is the desire and need for financial security. From the most recent work by His Holiness The Dalai Lama and Howard C. Cutler, M. D. we find that one-third of Americans view their pay checks as the prime motivation for working.[3] This view in itself is not unhealthy as most of us have expenses to meet and families to feed. The balance is tipped when the quest for money is pursued for the sake of making money itself. Individuals who follow this path suffer the pain of greed and find their efforts misplaced. The skewed focus on money is allowed to persist to the detriment of the family.

The more time spent at work, the less time there is to have with the family. Growing children especially need positive attention. When they fail to receive it they will act in ways to get the attention they need, though their actions may not always be positive. Everyone needs to receive positive attention and see themselves in good regard. Right Effort is what it takes to keep you mindful of the thoughts that come and go and the thoughts you choose to dwell on. Your job, in order to get your pain into a comfortable place, is to be the sentry of your mind's words. When you see a thought coming that is unproductive and unfruitful it is your responsibility to allow the thought to drop and not place any significant value on it. Such thoughts can be replaced by thoughts that will lead to less stress and fatigue.

When you are drained and stressed because of chronic pain it is your choice to remain focused on your thorn or to pay attention to the parts of you that are functioning well. If your right shoulder hurts all of the time or if chronic back pain is an issue, then do what you can to ease your pain. When you come to the place where you have done all that is possible and you have exhausted all that modern medicine can do then the responsibility to heal falls back into your court. Your muscles and joints may hurt and your eyes may be tired but at least you can see. Maybe you can get up and walk. You can possibly talk things over with a loved one or with a close friend. You can go out and give of yourself and help those who have greater needs than you.

By focusing on what works for you it is possible to decrease your suffering. When you dwell on the negative you end up not respecting yourself and dampen all possibility of pulling yourself out of your despair. In science there is a rule that states when you observe something the act of observation changes that which is observed. The same thing happens when you slow down enough to listen to your body and begin to take care of yourself. Practicing fearlessness in your observation of your pain will allow your pain to speak to you. You can not help but listen when you are quiet. It is as if your inner wisdom is activated and the body heals itself.

Instead of putting so much effort into doing it is much wiser to put greater effort into listening. In getting along in today's world it is important to have the ability to listen to others. When you listen to other's you gain their respect and they are more likely to listen to your point of view. It is also critical that you give yourself the opportunity to listen to yourself. Michael P. Nichols, Ph.D. tells us the following in his book, *The Lost Art of Listening: How Learning to Listen Can Improve Relationships*.

> "Anytime you demonstrate a willingness to listen with a
> minimum of defensiveness, criticism, or impatience, you are
> giving the gift of understanding- and earning the right to
> have it reciprocated."[4]

Pushing, striving, and rushing come with a price. That price is a loss of contact with your inner knowledge and wisdom. When you are fatigued and chronically exhausted you are less likely to listen to what others tell you and you are surely not going to clearly hear you own internal dialogue. We have all done things one way to later find out things didn't work out quite right and then told ourselves that we knew we should have proceeded another way. It comes down to attentive listening. There is no better way to discover your core beliefs than through the practice of meditation. Deeply hidden insights will reveal themselves at your prompting, but even this effort should be expended with an easy mind.

All yoga is not about standing on your head or holding your entire body weight up supported on your palms. Anything that brings the mind and the body into greater harmony is yoga. After years of pushing the body and forcing yourself to do things that you believed you had to do to survive, you might think that the last thing you need to do is get into something as strenuous as yoga. It might be that you have to take the first year of your yoga practice and do only restorative asanas. In these relaxing, restful poses you will set the stage for deeper listening. Your muscles and mind will come together and show you the way of ease.

The actual work or effort that will be required as you make serious inquiry into your beliefs will be in the realm of letting go. If things were easy to let go of then no one would ever have difficulty with the idea of dying. Some of us have a hard time letting go of stuff in our homes. How many times have you faced the need to get rid of an outdated article of clothing but kept putting it off because it had sentimental value. You know you can send it to the church or your favorite charity for their next fund raiser but you keep holding on to it. What is it that keeps you holding on? The same things keep us holding on to our old beliefs. When we open the door and quiet down enough to invite ourselves on the inward journey there will be beliefs you will find that you have ignored. There will be a great deal of emotional pain, regret for wrong choices, and blame. The effort here will be expended in the process of forgiveness.

Living unconsciously you are numb to the pain that has piled up over the years. You have ignored your body, have failed to exercise it and feed it properly. You have lifted too many heavy objects without listening to the messages that you own muscles have been sending you. As a result of this non-listening by the age of fifty, and sometimes younger, your body is riddled with arthritis. Bony overgrowths close the normal spaces between bones in an effort to protect that part of the body from further injury. You move your joints less and less in order to keep the pain at a minimum. By the time you're sixty you have a hard time getting up out of a chair because the quadriceps muscles, the muscles of the upper anterior thighs, have been allowed to atrophy.

In the beginning of a meditation practice you may find that things are moving along smoothly. After a few weeks you may start to get the hang of the meditation thing and begin to feel more calm and quiet. Over time, as you progress, you may find that your real issues begin to surface. This is when you have to make an effort to continue and cultivate the courage to remain gentle with yourself. There will be a tendency to blame yourself or others for all of the trials you have faced over the years. When these ideas begin to manifest it is wise to remain easy in mind and spirit. Be quick to forgive yourself and others.

When you find that the going starts getting rough this is the time to spend more time in restorative poses. Even in a restful pose there is a great deal of emotional activity going on. With awareness you will find that the movement of the breath will move muscle and fascia. As these places begin to shift, new visions and insights will arise. Listen to these insights and ask yourself what they mean for you. It will not always be an easy task but take it easy on yourself. You're only human and are not expected to be without mistakes.

In beginning a yoga practice your energy level will hopefully be high as you embark on a new adventure. The entire discipline of yoga is ahead of you and everything you read will be new to you. You will have what Shunryu Suzuki called beginner's mind.[5] Your goal will be to keep such an attitude alive as your practice matures. He tells us that we should practice with no attachment to results. If you are new to yoga and feel overwhelmed at all there is to learn, or if you are out of shape from years of neglect, or because of weight problems, then the following asana will assist in your restorative process. This pose is also helpful for those in intermediate and advanced practice when a plateau stage has been reached and there seems to be no way beyond it.

In this *asana*, as you direct yourself to release all effort, you will be taking the first steps toward emotional and physical recovery. The pose is referred to as Supported Child's Pose (*Salamba Balasana*). It is similar to *Uttassana* (Forward Bend) in that it is a calming, quieting, and restful posture. This is a

Supported child's pose

useful pose to assume if you find yourself waking up in the middle of the night or very early in the morning and your neck and or back is stiff. In the cooler winter months it will be cozier to cover yourself with a blanket as you rest in this place of comfort.

Start out by using a large cylindrical bolster or three to four blankets folded twelve inches wide. The blankets should be stacked neatly about as high as your hips would be while you are kneeling. Position the bolster between your legs and drop the torso to its resting place over the bolster. Let your arms be at your sides, with the palms facing down and adjacent to your ears. Turn the head to one side and sink into the bolster. Soften the belly and allow your exhalations to extend beyond their usual length. As you inhale through your nose fill the entire lung space and feel the expansion of the intercostal muscles and the separation of the ribs as the cleansing breath fills you. Sense any tension, tightness, or burning in your muscles of mastication (chewing muscles) as they maintain contact with the bolster. On the smooth, extended exhalation allow that sensation to dissipate into the bolster. After a few minutes turn your head to the opposite side and allow the contact with the bolster to show you were you need to release on this side. It may be that your sternocleidomastoid muscles (the anterior neck muscles) are tight. If so, feel the peak of their tension at the end of the inhalation and allow them to incrementally release with the even flow of the exhalation. Feel your entire being become one with the bolster as you trust your natural recuperative powers to engage and foster healing. Stay here for five to ten minutes or as long as your legs can tolerate the flexion that is required.

In order to get good at anything in life it takes time and effort. Time spent learning these postures and sitting in meditation with mindful effort will produce clarity of intention. This will lead to greater congruence in thought and action. Any sense of the lack of progress on your part will be a sign that work still needs to be done to master your listening skills. This is your body. Allow the channels of communication to open so that one part knows what the other part is doing and why. Direct your efforts towards acceptance of where you are right now, remain grounded and quiet so that you are not overcome by fear, and support those beliefs and ideas that bring ease while you put effort into being mindful of even your unwholesome thoughts. With time, practice, awareness, and intention they will eventually loosen their grip on you and you will experience greater freedom.

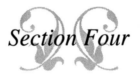

Section Four

CREATING SPACE

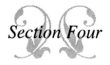

Section Four

CREATING SPACE

Introduction

*O*vercrowding creates tension. Social scientists like J.B. Calhoun demonstrated that rats raised in crowded conditions develop aggressive behaviors and some eventually die as a result of their stress.[1] Their thyroid glands produce increasing amounts of stress related hormone that eventually overwhelm their systems. The effects of social overcrowding in rodents can be used as an analogy relating to how thoughts are individually handled. The untrained mind is a potentially dangerous thing and can lead you down roads that not only increase suffering but also shorten your life.

For any of the one in fifty Americans who suffer from obsessive-compulsive disorder (OCD), the lack of space and overcrowding that occurs in their minds can be disabling. These individuals deal with excessive worries, doubts, and superstitious beliefs. Some of the common obsessions experienced by those suffering from OCD include fear of germs and dirt, fear of the loss of control of aggressive urges, excessive moral or religious doubt, and the need to have everything just right or always in its place. The common compulsions include repetitive hand washing, constant checking, counting, hoarding, and constant praying.[2]

When behavior patterns related to OCD interfere with daily life those individuals who are eventually diagnosed are usually treated with a class of drugs known as serotonin reuptake inhibitors. These drugs are none other than the commonly prescribed antidepressants of today: the Prozacs, Zolofts, Paxils, and Lexapros that are well known to the 6.3 million Americans daily ingesting them in their search for inner peace. Many individuals with phobias, such as agoraphobia or the fear of "open spaces" may also take the same class of drugs. Agoraphobics are afraid of experiencing the feelings of panic. Up to 40 million Americans suffer from some type of phobia. That number approaches 900 million worldwide.

If you live with pain on a daily basis you probably also suffer from agliophobia or odyneophobia. Both refer to the fear of pain. Pain causes you to close down around it in your attempt to keep it below the level of consciousness. Unfortunately this behavior is unsustainable and pain rears its ugly head with a greater vengeance, causing the cycle of pain and fear to feed on each other at your expense. You end up investing precious energy trying to keep pain under control and lose out on activities that would have otherwise resulted in joy and fulfillment. No wonder anger is a constant sidekick.

In taking the first steps in developing a meditation practice, or making a commitment to deepen your practice, you will find issues intensifying. Bringing your problems to the front burner and intentionally turning up the heat takes courage. Some are motivated to begin by the realization that pain has taken over and has come to rule their life. Things become so uncomfortable that something must be done. This is actually a good thing, though it doesn't make it any easier.

The following chapters will lead you into the meditative mode in a way that promotes the expansion of consciousness. Moving ahead with gentleness, and a somewhat playful attitude of exploration, allow yourself to experience that which you have feared in the past. As you proceed, direction will be given on how to use your breath as an anchor. This will keep you grounded and direct you away from panic situations. With serious practice you will find there is more space and potential than you ever thought possible.

Physical, emotional, and spiritual rewards are waiting to be discovered. As you learn to lighten you heart and develop greater appreciation for past experiences you will discover their true value to your path. As you improve your ability to drop into the stillness around you an internal shift will occur as the process of dissolution of past trauma proceeds. Releasing past unwholesome beliefs as insight grows permits your inner beauty to blossom. You will find life more to your liking as mind, body, and spirit come into alignment and as your capacity to generate love, hope, joy, peace, and compassion blooms.

As space opens up your real priorities will make themselves known and you will have the wisdom to move in the direction of their manifestation. Learning more about yourself and about others will bring you to a place of greater patience, yet at the same time, you will know how to exercise greater determination, persistence, endurance, and courage. You will find yourself expressing higher levels of personal responsibility in all aspects of your life as you unearth a new sense of confidence and conviction.

Bringing your practice to a different level, with the companionship of this inner strength and compassion, may lead you to begin a practice of *tonglen*. The word *tonglen* means "taking in and sending out."[3] This courageous form of meditation practice will allow you to expand your level of giving to others as well as yourself. It will allow you to feel what is really going on and experience unshielded with an open heart. As you move forward, I encourage you to come back to your practice daily and know that your work is important.

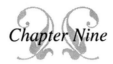

Chapter Nine

Deeper Meditation

*L*ike everything else in life you attract the things that are most dominant in your mind. Through a natural progression, a morning meditation routine will arise when right effort is applied. Once you realize your responsibility in creating the space for a meditation practice and drop the idea that you will get to it when you have more time, things begin to happen. Chronic physical discomfort or the unsatisfactory way you deal with daily demands and interruptions may finally reach a kindling point and prod you to seriously start your inner work. In a short time, as you experience a small degree of success, it is natural to want to experience more of the same. The great thing about life is that as you move along obtaining the results that you want to see, the easier it is to replicate your result.

In moving deeper into a meditation practice there will be times when the going is no longer easy. The goal is not to replicate anything but to be open and make internal space for whatever it is that has to come up for you. Old harmful emotions like anger, jealousy, and greed will arise. It is easy to justify why you would want to wallow in these states and not let them go. Ego finds it hard to open up and see any other side of the story. In your quite space it is necessary to stand beside ego, watch it's mechanism of action and not get pulled into its line of limited thinking.

As you sit and watch your thoughts, in order to separate yourself from their energy, it is useful to start by labeling them. As you take an in-breath and become aware of a thought developing simply label the thought "thinking." This is not a far fetched idea as thoughts are just thinking. Instead of following your usual story-line to its end you break the pattern and well-worn habit by calling the thought just what it is. Nothing extra is added. Do not get lost in its content; simply put a name on the process. When you sit and find a problem issue arises, be it work related or personal, apply the label "thinking" and continue following your breath.

Once a thought is labeled, on the out-breath, just think dissolve. Any desire or impulse to grasp and hold on to the thought is allowed to drop. Let the thought and any connection you have to it melt into the great unknown. You are intentionally making space to safely release any grasping tendencies you have. It is a time to empty and though this release sounds simple, it takes a great deal of courage and trust to let go of long held ideas and beliefs.

To just let go and be with emptiness can be difficult because it means that you allow yourself to give up all ideas of who and what you think you are. It is a foreign concept to suggest letting go of ideas because of the attachments developed over the years. Everyone is grasping. There are wants for more money, better looks, more friends, an easier job, and a bigger house. The human mind always wants more. It is the way that it has been programmed. Our ideas as a society as to what are considered necessities has changed over time. In 1970, 20% of Americans felt that a second car was a necessity. In the year 2000, that number rose to 59%. Similarly, thirty years ago, 3% felt that a second television set was necessary versus 45% in 2000.[1] Status and the acquisition of wealth with its attendant "stuff," have become synonymous with the state of happiness. Such ideas, instead of allowing for the creation of more space in one's life, simply end up cluttering lives as well as our planet.

For many reasons, the switch has been thrown and everyone believes that in order to be someone you have to be wealthy. The focus has been misplaced and centers on externals. How many times have you said, "I'll be happy when I get _____?" You fill in the blank. Humans do not need things to be fulfilled. They need to be doing the things that they love, the things that allow them to express the passion within. The reality of life is that we are complete already. It is something that has long been forgotten. In the process of socialization we have become needier in many ways.

Yoga and meditation will show you the way back to your real self with its real needs. The spaces between the breath and between your thoughts are filled with wisdom.

Isn't it time to give yourself the gift of getting to know yourself. Author and cultural critic, Bell Hooks reminds us that the goal is not to become pain free but to "restore a sense of balance that will allow us to cope with our pain in ways that are restorative. So pain isn't perceived as the enemy but as the point of possibility and transformation."[2]

Moving into meditation may seem like you are going deeper into your own self-centeredness, but the goal is to see your attachment to self and cultivate the courage to gently break the connection. If you have never tried sitting with yourself to meditate I offer the promise that you will learn many things about yourself by putting in some small chunks of time and some effort. Like everything else, it will take time and experience to truly benefit, but once you start and make up your mind to work with a daily meditation practice you will have wondered why it took you so long to start in the first place. There will be a sense of struggle at first as you become more acutely aware of you habitual thought processes. You need not worry about doing it right because there is no real right way or wrong way.

There are many varieties of meditation. One kind does not fit all but one of the more popular schools of meditation is exemplified by the Insight Meditation Society in Barre, Massachusetts. The center was founded in 1975 by Sharon Salzberg, Joseph Goldstein, and Jack Kornfield. Insight meditation or *vipassana* is the practice of moment to moment mindfulness. This type of meditation is taught in the Theravada tradition of Buddhism as taught by the Buddha over 2500 years ago. In such teachings, as in all of the teachings of the Buddha, we learn that suffering is part of life. As we deepen our practice we find that attachment to ideas, beliefs, results, and objects result in suffering because of their impermanence. The way out of suffering is through the release of all attachment. In getting over our need to prove anything we experience what is pure and real in this moment.

Insight meditation is about coming back to the moment. In your silence, which is not really silence, as we all have a constant internal dialogue, the one constant is your breath. It acts like an anchor. As long as you are alive the breath will be with you. When practicing insight meditation we capitalize on this fact. On the other hand, thoughts will come and go. They repeat themselves and jump all over the place in a seemingly disorganized manner. By following your breath you find that you can center yourself and more easily watch the thoughts come and go without attachment.

Another tip to think about when just starting a meditation practice is while following the breath do not force or hold the breath. Give up any desire to try to control the breath. Let it flow naturally and observe that some breaths will be long and deep while others will be short and shallow. When this awareness arises, simply label the breath as "long" or "short." In the beginning do not concern yourself with manipulating the breath. That will come later when you get into the practice of pranayamma. At the start just observe the breath and let it do what it wants to.

The same holds true for your thoughts. There is no need to try to control your thoughts. When you tell yourself that you have to control your thoughts they get wilder and you end up calling yourself a failure. Your job is to observe and watch the patterns. When you find yourself lost in a storyline gently notice that, label the thoughts as "thinking," and on the out-breath let everything dissolve. It takes concentration and awareness but by practicing this on a daily basis both will improve and you will discover greater clarity in you day to day activities.

Another way to practice using the breath is to count as you inhale or exhale. You may choose to count before each in-breath. The idea is to count just before taking the breath and not during the movement of the breath. It is reasonable to count for a total of ten breaths then start over. If you lose track, notice that fact and start again. Once you have done this for three or four cycles you can change and make your count at the end of the exhalation. During the inhalation and exhalation keep the mind focused on the sensation of the breath as it moves through the nasal passages. A good point of *dristi*, or concentration, is at the tip of the nose, feeling the point of contact between the movement of air and the mucosal lining of the nasal passages. When your mind wanders to other parts of your body, such as the abdomen as it rises with each in-breath, bring your attention back to the point of contact in the nose. Just as a comfortable speed for a runner to take is one that allows him to speak simultaneously, so should you work with your breath in a state of ease. There is no need to get intense over this or any exercise. If there is any cogwheel or ratchet-like movement of the breath observe this phenomenon. It will smooth out with practice and intention.

The best tone of voice that I have heard through reading has been that of Thich Nhat Hanh. Read a few pages of one of his many books and you will quickly get the idea of how best to talk to yourself on these self-guided journeys. His voice is authoritative yet comforting, sure yet gentle, but most of all it is kind and understanding. You understand more about your life than anyone else. It is when you think that you have to prove your existence to others or yourself that you lose contact with your inner voice. When you continue to listen to internal tapes from the past you are not truly doing what you want to be doing or moving to live your purpose. Removing any harsh self-criticism is key to finding inner peace. As you undertake these deeper meditations you will need to begin the practice of forgiveness. You will have to learn how to take it easy on yourself.

Sharon Salzberg, who was mentioned above, has written a book devoted to the practice of being kind to others as well as yourself. The book is titled *Loving-Kindness: The Revolutionary Art of Happiness.*[3] In her book she expounds on the benefits of meditation most notably developing a greater connection to others. By cultivating skillful minds one comes to realize that it is impossible to be angry and kind at the same time. One learns that it is beneficial to drop those unskillful actions and beliefs that lead to further suffering and replace them with actions and thoughts that reflect appreciation for who you are in relation to others. You and the other are one thus everyone including yourself deserves kindness.

With all of the childhood hurts we sustain, we harden. We tighten up and shut down. We unknowingly close ourselves off from our own goodness and the goodness of others. We get to a place where we think we know what the results will be of any and all actions we take. In assuming many things, nothing is new, and we lose our spontaneity. We become like robots incapable of feeling, incapable of dealing with human emotions, ours or those of others. We may try to fix things but we don't know how to feel the suffering of others. We lack compassion and thus cut ourselves off from others because we are afraid of getting tied up in their problems. We figure we have enough of our own problems to deal with and who needs more burdens.

The problem is that when we cut ourselves off from others we tend to operate from a position of fear. It is only when we allow ourselves to remain open to the trials and tribulations of others that we can feel connected and whole. By exercising compassion for others we are able to transfer that compassion to ourselves. Pema Chodron explains the practice of *tonglen*, in her book *Start Where You Are: A Guide to Compassionate Living*.[4] She also starts out with the premise that everyone has basic goodness. No matter what anger, doubt, fear, or hatred you may feel, there is always an underlying goodness within.

In the practice of *tonglen*, the usual human desire to avoid painful and unpleasant emotions is turned upside down. In this style of meditation you begin by acknowledging that you are angry or jealous. You also recognize that at any given moment there are millions of other individuals in our world experiencing these exact same emotions. With courage you intentionally breathe in these feelings that others are living so that they no longer have them. With the out breath you put out your wish that everyone including yourself would be free of such suffering.

In both loving-kindness meditation and *tonglen* there is the connection to innate goodness. It is expressed continually in the affirmations with the former type of meditation and given away to others in the latter. It is useful to start with loving-kindness meditation and develop your skills and later move on to *tonglen* as it requires greater confidence, courage, and commitment.

LOVING-KINDNESS MEDITATION

In your quiet place, sitting comfortably with the attitude of royalty, begin to gently focus on the movement of your breath as it washes over the inner lining of the nasal passages. As extraneous sounds come into your awareness acknowledge them and let them slip away from focus. Feeling yourself moving into your center begin to broaden your physical and mental space by remaining grounded and picturing the expanse of the ocean or the continual outward spread of our expanding universe.

There will be areas of your body where you will experience a pulling sensation, or burning, squeezing, or tightness. These are the places you have closed down from past physical or emotional trauma. At some point you felt it was necessary to protect yourself from a perceived threat and your response was to tighten. This may be an area of chronic nagging pain or it may be only noticeable when you begin to slow down and relax at the end of the day or end of the work week. Because you know that you need to keep going you have decided to ignore your pain. It is as if you had no other choice.

Recognize and feel as much of this pain as you comfortably can before the urge to withdrawal pulls you back. Listen to the pain and allow your body and muscularature to minutely shift as it is directed by the breath. Allow the movement of the breath, using the energy of the pain, to create more physical space between the joints and muscles you are working with. For example, if you are concentrating on cervical neck pain let both the inhalation and the exhalation bring your entire spine into a longer configuration. Trust that the large paraspinal muscles on either side of your spine will wake up and respond to your intention and do their job more effectively thus creating greater space between your head and your pelvis. Feel the sternum or breastbone rise and your shoulders and chest broaden without ballooning out as the breath is allowed to make space where before there had only been tightness and constriction.

As you expand yet remain grounded, start to suggest to yourself the following:

- ☯ I am filled with love and compassion for myself and others
- ☯ I am peace
- ☯ Love, joy, and understanding fill my being
- ☯ I deserve forgiveness
- ☯ I accept myself where I am right now
- ☯ I am the picture of health and wholeness
- ☯ Just as a flower blooms without effort, so shall I

Bask in the comfort these words bring. Feel free to create affirmations of your own that are more to your liking or that have a better fit for your situation. Sit with these ideas for five or ten minutes and realize that you can come back to them no matter what you are involved in the rest of the day. You can suggest to yourself that every time you pick up a pen or every time you answer the phone you will remind yourself of these messages and allow yourself to feel their reality.

When doubt or fear enters your mind realize that it is the ego's way of trying to keep things the way they are. You have a choice as to where you place your attention and the sooner you begin the work of developing a skillful mind, the sooner you will begin to reap the benefits. As you practice allow your mind to drop into your open heart as you experience deeper levels of insight, understanding, and compassion.

TONGLEN PRACTICE

As you advance in your practice and find that you wish to deepen your experience you may want to try *tonglen*. As mentioned above it incorporates loving-kindness techniques but adds the intention that the work is being done not only for you but for all who suffer. Again, center yourself as much as possible with the initial insight breathing. As you count the breaths feel your attention move inward. Allow yourself to open and touch your basic goodness. As an area of pain or tightness in your body comes into awareness let your mind recognize that sensation as deeply as possible. In touch with your pain bring to mind a loved one who currently has a painful condition. Breath in your pain and their pain as you affirm the following: may they be free from suffering and may they know the root of happiness.

At first, this part of the meditation may seem difficult to do because you feel you have to be willing to take on more pain than you already have. The truth is that you are exposed to pain and suffering more than you are aware of. Look at how many times you watch the TV news, read the newspaper, or listen to the radio about the war in Iraq or about the mother with the postpartum depression who kills her two children. As long as these terrible events are happening to someone else you feel semi-safe but they affect your mind, body, and spirit on a very deep level. You begin to think how can someone murder their own child or how can you ever board an airliner without suspicion? Long after hearing such news your mind goes back to thinking of the shattered, ruined, and lost lives. You know pain even though it scares you. Put the fear aside and look at the raw pain. It is the only way to make friends with it. Practicing this way desensitizes you of the usual fear surrounding adversity.

Once connected with your pain and that of your beneficiary, on the out breath affirm freedom from pain for all living beings, including your loved one and yourself. This will encompass even those you don't know and will never know and allows your compassion to spread and grow. In a single day over 200,000 people starve to death, with 826 million individuals worldwide remaining chronically hungry. Poverty is rampant with almost half (2.8 billion) of the world population living on less than two dollars a day.[5] The fact that someone in the world commits suicide every forty seconds is a testament to just how great the suffering is.

As you develop more proficiency you can do *tonglen* for those individuals who give you a hard time during your work day. As an encounter occurs and difficult emotions arise, you can silently perform your practice right on the spot, breathing in the difficulty as you wish for your adversary to have peace and joy, then sending out the same goodwill to everyone who is suffering in the same manner. Family members also act as a good source of material to work with as they always know just what buttons to push to get your dander up.

In the practice of *tonglen* you sit and take in all of the suffering of the world but it is done with your experience of great space. In sitting you identify a difficult situation in your life and realize that there are millions of people in the world dealing with a similar or worse situation. Take that in and on the out-breath you give away all of the good and all of the joy that you know, but also give it to yourself. You have come to a place where you are willing to share all that you have with others. This kind of meditation takes you away from the habitual way of thinking that we all have of wanting only those things that are pleasurable and avoiding those things that cause suffering. As Pema says, "This is advanced practice." She also says that everyone can do it.

At the start of a meditation practice it is ideal to sit for twenty minutes twice a day sitting the first thing in the morning and just before going to bed. The use of a meditation pillow (the *zafu*) and a cushion (the *zabuton*) help align pelvis and the spine for the posture most conducive to comfortable sitting. The pelvis should be tilted forward so that you are sitting on the ischial tuberosities or the sit bones and the lower spine has its normal lordotic curve (the low back curves inward toward the abdomen). Different schools of thought exist concerning whether the eyes should remain open or closed. In the way of Shambala training, such as the school of mind training as practiced by Pema Chodron, it is recommended to keep the eyes open. This way it is easier to stay in touch with where you are and it is more difficult to fall asleep. In other types of meditation it is taught to keep the eyes gently closed thus keeping the focus inward. Find what works for you and do not be concerned if you move between methods as your needs will change from time to time.

To believe that the goal of a meditative state is to achieve bliss is an inaccurate idea of what meditation is. Meditation is more an intention to spend time with yourself and your thoughts, whatever they may be. It is a willingness to sit still and watch what is going on in your mind in an effort to learn more intimately the methods of the mind. To sit, watch, and remain non-reactive as the mind grasps for something to hold on to leads to the fruits of enlightenment. When you begin your practice it is like turning up the volume on a radio that is tuned between two stations. There is a great deal of static and only occasionally can you sense clarity.

With training, the mind will go everywhere and anywhere. When you make the effort to sit you will find that not all of your thoughts are noble. You will face the contrast of the idealized picture you have of yourself and the real you. Everyone tends to view themselves in a good light using rationalization to negate any thoughts or actions that might be seen as selfish or self-centered. Acting and thinking as if asleep you may not even be aware of your projection of self-centeredness. With a persistent practice you will become more aware of your motives and the motives of others. In closer contact with your thoughts and emotions it is easier to call up the courage to identify your fearful states. It will be more natural to pull up the inner strength that will help you successfully through any difficult situation and you will do it with grace.

Sitting in meditation is not going to always bring that blissful, peaceful state that you see in pictures. It will bring you peace at times and turbulence at other times. The goal is to find what the Buddhists describe as the middle way. The healthy life is the life of balance. Not too much excitement and not too much peace, but somewhere in the middle. It is one thing to be a workaholic and another thing to be a bum. Neither condition is healthy. The middle way naturally brings balance and satisfaction.

It will be necessary for you to make the time to meditate. It may mean that you have to get up ten minutes earlier and go to bed ten minutes later, but eventually you may find the time you spend in meditation to be more restorative than your restless sleep. In the beginning you may believe that it would be wonderful to be able to meditate all day long thinking that your day of enlightenment will arrive sooner. You may eventually become angry over the fact that you cannot meditate five or six hours a day and think that if you could just be like a monk or hermit and be alone in a cave that you would find your truth without haste. As the practice matures you will realize what hard work it would be to meditate for hours at a time. Your legs would fall asleep after a short time, your back will hurt and the scary stuff that no one wants to look at would get overwhelming. There is a middle way in meditation and with time and practice you will find it.

A focused meditative state is more wakeful than the usual waking state. You will learn that you can carry that state with you into difficult and challenging issues at work and at home. In the tough moments you can rely on your breath to center yourself. You can consciously ground yourself when the energy of others is going wild all around you. When you are rushed and pushed to the limit by the needs of others you can open your heart, elongate your spine, plant your feet on the ground and breathe. You do not have to sigh or force your breath. Use the easy movement of the breath and the sensation of its coolness as it enters your physical body to temper the flames of rustled emotions. These simple actions remind you that you are bigger than the situation you find yourself in and you will be able to proceed with minimal suffering.

Sitting on the mat you never know what is going to come up. Dropping all expectations and remaining open to whatever comes up allows for greater exploration and makes room for the bigger picture to appear. The world and our lives are full of suffering. Meditation offers you a safe haven to look at the stuff that scares and frightens you. These are the demons that you choose to ignore in your daily life by way of self-imposed distractions. The trash has to be taken out. The laundry needs to be done. That report has to be completed. The next episode of the Soprano's is on. There are always things to do that will keep you occupied and away from the solitude that can make you whole. Many folks are afraid to spend time with themselves letting the TV keep them company. The latest best-selling novel keeps them in suspense and turning the page for a story when the greatest story we will ever know, if we give ourselves a chance, is our own story.

Everyone has a different point where they say that enough is enough. There is great variability in the tolerance individuals display when it comes to being comfortable with the condition of their lives. What will it take for you to take a closer look? The pain that you are trying to rid yourself of is the wake up call to look deeper. It is asking you to ask yourself what is wrong. Where are your thinking and expectations so out of line that you suffer daily at the cost of living a fulfilling life? How long will you continue to allow yourself to be held prisoner by your pain?

Today is all that you have. No one is guaranteed the next breath. This breath may well be your last. Not that this is a bad thing but this knowledge can serve to wake you up to start enjoying and appreciating what is right in front of you while living minute to minute with greater awareness. You can learn to prioritize and let the insignificant stuff fall by the wayside. It can be fun getting to know yourself. Why settle for an idealized picture of who you are when you can allow yourself to unfold and live to your full potential if you would only look deeper?

Sitting in meditation the roots of your feeling will emerge. You will find why you have been angry over certain events in your life and through practice develop compassion and forgiveness concerning the anger. You will find your source of energy shifting from a hot burning consuming energy, the energy of anger, to a cool calm steady source of peaceful energy. In Chinese medicine terms your energy source will shift from the liver to the calmer kidney chi. Insights will arise that will bring resolution and new beginnings but it won't happen in a day. Fear will try to come back at you each day but with your new found wisdom you will see it for what it is. It may not even happen in a year but over time you will begin to laugh at it and make jest of it as you settle into a new comfort zone.

There is a law in science that tells us when we observe something the simple act of observation changes it. By observing yourself in meditation you change yourself. The body and mind know how to heal as long as we get out of the way. Meditation allows the healing to occur naturally. You will cry, you will ache, you will not get all of the answers that you wanted, but you will change. Others will notice that change and begin to inquire about it. At that point you can share your story. People will open up to you.

Meditation may seem like a lonely time but there is so much going on inside that it is anything but lonely. In those peak times during meditation you will know that you are one with everything; one with the leaves on the trees outside of your window, one with the clouds and their water droplets, one with the thunder, and one with the lightening. With that feeling of one-ness comes the ability to accept that which is otherwise unacceptable. Disruptive and crude behavior in others is now understood and their roots become perfectly clear. The benefits of past bad experiences rise as new insight. Meaning becomes evident. Past hurts heal. Sit long enough and they will explain themselves to you in a clear voice. You will be your own best friend and the friend of others.

What part of your body is crying out for attention? Where is it that you are feeling pain on a daily basis? Where is the pain that wakes you up at night? Sitting will show you the thoughts and beliefs that keep you holding on to your pain. This holding on is an attempt to keep yourself from know-ing your pain. It keeps you away from being able to see clearly. It keeps you in a fog about who you are and what you can do to experience life more fully.

When you come to a place where you actually feel and see your wall there is where the work begins. You may feel that you will never figure out what is going on in that place. You tell yourself that there is no way in this lifetime that you will ever have the time nor the energy to figure out the complexities of thoughts, feelings and emotions that are intermixing to make you feel what you are feeling. You feel overwhelmed by the experiences that come back to haunt you. This is where kindness and gentleness come in to play but it is difficult to be kind and gentle in a place where so much frustration, so much anger, is stored and concentrated. It is held in a mistaken effort for self-protection. Yes, such holding on does protect you. It protects your ego that thinks you need to be a certain way, but that protection also keeps you from knowing your true power.

Everyone has fear but not everyone knows fear. Are you willing to know fear? Are you willing to look at your own fears to see what it is that you're trying to protect yourself from? Are you ready to drop your ideas of who you think you are and see what happens? It is risky but it is all that we were meant to do. Why is it that we all make it so hard on ourselves? To soften and sit with our pain and frustration we sit in meditation, wait for the wall to appear, and then courageously continue to sit. When the impulse arises to squeeze a jaw muscle or tighten a neck flexor, see the impulse and gently let it pass. You do not have to react to every impulse that comes up. In the busy day to day stuff that comes up we usually tighten up and move forward. In meditation we allow ourselves to sit without reacting and let the scene play through without getting tight inside and closing down.

Confronted with your internal wall you may feel you have traveled to the end of the road. There you find a thousand-foot granite rock. The giant rock takes the shape of a colossal –U- and you've meandered right into the center of it. You can turn around and go back but knowing what that's like it's not an option. You can decide to stay in the –U- for as long as you can. Up against the rock you begin to see things: things that bother you, things that make you tense. These are your demons. These are the thoughts of inadequacy, feelings of unworthiness and lack, feelings of separateness and aloneness.

What can you do to allow yourself to stay there for a while and not criticize yourself, and not judge past behaviors and actions? You can walk up to the huge rock and gently touch it. You can physically and emotionally connect with the rock and experience it for what it is. It is there and you are there. You are not the rock but you believe that it is in your way. Will that rock stay there forever? On first impression looking at and feeling it you believe the only thing that could move that rock is dynamite. You can't use dynamite because you're standing right there with the rock. So you conclude that, no, there is nothing that will move that rock.

There is a vacation spot in western North Carolina called Linville Falls. A short walk from the parking lot will get you to the falls. It is a quiet, cool walk, with a 3-4% grade that will bring you to a resting place where you can sit on the rocks and watch the water make its way effortlessly downhill. There are a number of small, shallow pools where the water moves slowly. Looking there you see bathers submerged in the cool water with their heads resting on the sand or a towel placed on a small rock. Ten to fifteen minutes of sitting will bring you closer to nature as your inner stillness broadens. The water, the rocks, and the trees are no longer separate objects but become part of you.

Walking a little further there are larger falls where the rocks are bigger and the water moves with greater force. The terrain twists and turns as the water rumbles down dropping into successive pools until it opens into an expansive pool just below the scenic overlook. You could follow the pool and watch the water make its way around the curving rock. Looking over a walled ledge to the other side is a deep drop where the speed and intensity of the falling water is animated and wild. The water eventually floods into a dark underground hole traveling deep into the earth.

Turning back to look upstream you notice plaques bolted onto the rocks. They describe the geological changes that occurred in the falls over the past ten to twelve million years. Ten million years ago this very place sat fifteen miles upstream. It boarders inconceivable to think that all of that rock could move that far, but the power of time, the power of the water, and the constant changes that occur in the geological make-up of the earth took place moment by moment. The change occurred so slowly that on a daily basis it appeared that nothing had changed or that nothing would ever change. But from a prospective of twelve million years, the change was unbelievable.

It is not that we have twelve million years to change or that we want to wait that long for our change to occur but we have to open our senses and realize that we do change all of the time. This realization alone could be enough to see each of us though our most difficult times. Meditation will act like a magnifying glass and augment the minute changes that always occur in the mind and body and allow you to be privy to the wonders within. Go deeper.

Chapter Ten

Time for Healing

*G*entleness, kindness, openness, softness, these are the words that come to mind when we want healing to take place. When things go wrong and pile up like smelly compost it is second nature to look for someone to blame. Though it may be the easy way out, such action will not lead to the resolution of suffering. Finding someone or some event to blame for your problems allows you to overlook the fact that your buttons have been pushed. Blame says it not your fault or your doing, but something beyond your control has power over you and victim mentality takes over.

I have two sons, nine and four years old. The issue of blame comes up multiple times a day. As soon as Joel, the youngest, starts crying, John Trey will yell, "I didn't do anything." He is conditioned that he will take the blame. Many times Joel will start crying because his big brother was playing too rough with him. We encourage John Trey to take it easy on his brother but we also take into account that John Trey is just a youngster and has his own learning curve. Learning to take responsibility in small doses is important. The same holds for moving into mindfulness. Such a move should be taken in incremental steps otherwise trying to take on too much at once will lead to disappointment and blame. Though we are all well beyond nine years old and presumably should know better it is so easy to blame. It is time to bring our bodies and minds in line with the emotions. This is the first step in healing.

In mindfulness training it is critical to assume a gentle posture when dealing with your sense of blame. If you can't find someone to be responsible for your predicament the next step of turning on yourself is a prescription for disaster. Start beating yourself up and everyone around you suffers. The problem starts when, as a child, you were assigned blame by a parent who also received blame. Until you are able to make that connection you will pass blame on to your children. The cycle will continue until you decide to question where these behaviors came from. Pain and discomfort are your teachers and tutors. They will wake you up. Meditations on forgiveness and kindness will come in useful as a way to break the self-defeating patterns acquired in your formative years.

In a child's world everything revolves around him. All that happens, good and bad, is understood as a result of their doing. Parents divorce and the child feels responsible, continuing to carry that responsibility until they are taught otherwise. I encourage you to look back in meditation and see how many events in your life you are still holding this way. As you identify these painful memories gently encourage and reassure yourself with the explanation that in an imperfect world, painful events will happen to everyone. The guilt is real but was imposed by the child mind that still sees itself as a child, unaware of the now responsible adult. This inner undoing takes a great deal of patience but as you become more patient with yourself new understanding will spill over into your relationships and your joy will multiply.

A seemingly benign series of events cumulatively contributed to who you are today. These events, bothering you for years, creating stress and tension in your life, made you feel responsible for things that were beyond your control. The courageous first step is to own your own stuff, take responsibility for where you are and begin to realize that outside events alone are not what make you angry. It is your internal reaction to what has transpired that burns you up and eats at your core. You may blame your partner for your anger believing that you are being asked to do something you don't want to do. The reality may be that you fear confrontation and speaking your mind, exposing your feelings, will leave you vulnerable. When you see the real issues you act from a place of authenticity, coming from center, with your words and actions in agreement.

As you progressively develop the courage to accept more responsibility you have to ask, how can you appreciate the multitude of ways you have cared for yourself in the past? What forgotten choices, that you never gave yourself credit for, were made that brought you to where you are today? Obviously you have done something right to still be here today. No matter how bad you think your situation is, especially in comparison to someone you believe is better off, you have chosen, on a daily basis, those things that have allowed you to survive. In the business of living we have lost touch with our past adaptive actions. We have downplayed these essential adaptive actions. These choices and actions were necessary for continued survival. Take the time to appreciate your unique situation and your individual way of dealing with the perceived and real dangers that you face on a daily basis.

We all learn patterns of behavior as children. Without acknowledging that young personality within, for all that it has done, you do a disservice to yourself. Graciously thank that person within and learn to ask what you can do for yourself. Soften just enough to sense that there is more to you right now than what you think there is. Stop long enough to feel your own presence. If you do, you will find the freedom that you have been seeking. It is now present and always has been.

A frightened young child of seven or eight, when faced with an overwhelming situation, will many times stand there and take it. The primitive internal response is to freeze, taking neither flight nor fight. Fear of feeding into the other person's energy leaves you standing there defenseless as the event unfolds and eventually diffuses. There is a down side to utilizing a frozen state as a coping mechanism. It is an inability to deal with what is happening in the moment. When the mind and body remain frozen the price to pay is chronic neck pain, unresolved anger and a generally depressed attitude.

If you are currently in your forties or fifties chances are high that you were a victim of corporal punishment. In the 1950's ninety-nine percent of parents supported its use as a disciplinary mode. Things have improved to a degree but even today up to fifty percent of parents still support its use.[1] Such abuse left you feeling weak and defenseless. These feelings do not just go away with age. They persist and cloud everything you do. They affect your expectations of yourself and others.

Reading self-help books only goes so far. There is real work that has to be done and it takes an inner strength that you are not familiar with. To find that strength you need to go to inner places that you have not dared to venture up until now. To see the path clearly the weeds have to be burned and pulled. One way of proceeding is to try and force this new way of thinking upon yourself and pay with greater resistance in the future. This simply delays your pain. Another way is to begin appreciating where you are today no matter how terrible your situation is. Even if it takes all of your effort to be thankful for your next breath it is healthier to move into this space than stay in the painful state you are now in.

It is easy to be thankful and grateful when there is no pain. It is another thing to be grateful when pain waits for you in the morning even before you open your eyes, follows you throughout the day, and then tucks you into bed at night for a restless sleep. In quiet mediation it is possible to touch your pain. It is possible to begin to look at your anger from a distance. As you become more familiar with it you learn to identify what thoughts trigger it and make it grip you tighter. Over time and with much practice you can learn to diffuse it and transform it into a positive force. Your anger and your pain are the bullies of your world. It will take creative thinking and action to deal with them. New insights will come to you as you listen with a tuned ear while in meditation. As you sit, ask what it is today that you can be thankful for?

Painful emotions are the last thing in the world that anyone wants to deal with but your choices are to let things remain the way they are and continue to put up with your pain or make the move to face it and be willing to make some mistakes and live with them for the short time that it will take you to make further corrective action. This is the element that we seem to forget. Things are always changing and you have more input into how they change than you are aware of. Your power has been taken away by ignorance of right action and right effort. You simply did not know any better. Now there is a chance to change all of that but you must do the work.

You have not known what to do so you persisted in doing the same thing over and over with the same painful results. Now is the time to be thankful for all that has gone before you. Every past hurt can be viewed as a message to awaken to your own power. Touching the pain in gratitude is a way of awakening compassion making you raw enough to feel what others have felt. Opening your heart and allowing it to soften makes way for new opportunity to serve others. In the process of serving others you deepen your appreciation for what you have faced along your path. Instead of trying to get out of the way of life, stepping back, and trying to get out of the range of pain, you need to move into your pain.

Right now you have your back up against the wall, hands in tight fists, face buried deep in bent arms, and back hunched forward to protect your heart. Life passes you by as you stand there in a futile attempt at self protection. What is it that is actually hurting you? Can you open enough to get a glimpse that it might be your need to feel safe in a scary world. To heal you have to be willing to see what is really going on. You have to be able to see cause and effect and know that you are part of the decision tree. Even though you do not want to be in this situation it is necessary to acknowledge the fact that you are in order to move into a new place. Trying to wish things away or trying to be a tougher person will not work.

In your listening you may be led to seek further medical advice. It is probable that up until now you lacked the trust in others to help you. Fear of the unknown or horror stories from others may have to be overlooked as you build trust in healthcare professionals. If you have been undergoing long term therapy with no obvious beneficial results it may be time to thank your current provider and seek other opinions. Have you been ignoring the prompting of loved ones to seek other help? If so, ask yourself why you are resisting and examine your fear. Next take the steps to get done what needs to be done. The love you receive from your spouse, family, and friends may be just what it takes to get you over the edge and moving toward healing.

It is time to replace stubbornness and independence with trust and openness. If you have been trying for years to get relief and seem only to be get-

165

ting worse outside help is needed. Internal messages are repeated with lack of awareness of their power over you. You will need honest input from objective sources to pull you away from old habitual circular thinking. Stay open in your meditation and answers will come as you grow in appreciation of your new willingness to do what you have to do to feel better.

As you begin to appreciate yourself just as you are with pain, weakness, and that washed out feeling, and accept the help that you need your confidence will grow. You will find yourself moving toward the things you want but had put off because of lack of energy. The displaced energy previously expended in maintaining a tough exterior is now available for your desired activities. Your pain and discomfort may be more acute as you begin to drop your defenses. You will feel overwhelmed but appreciating this as part of the process reinforces the idea that you have chosen to move toward health and balance. You are ready for healing.

As you continue to meditate, and get the help that you need, you will discover new strengths. Just as a child needs to be allowed to win when playing, you need small victories. In your tangled emotional state the conditioned self has overlooked the small victories you accomplish daily. If you go to work, provide for your family, and serve to the best of your ability then it is healthy to feel positive about this. On the other hand if you are disabled secondary to your illness and you choose to take the first steps at appreciating your current condition this is also very positive. Your willingness to feel your pain in this new light will not be missed by those around you. As you open to your plight others will open up and make deeper connections with you. The sense of dependency will slowly dissolve as you reclaim your power and any sense of weakness will be viewed as a potential for strength. This all transpires through the benefits of appreciation.

The work now is to go back to the young child within and acknowledge what a great job he did in coping with all of the difficult situations doing what he could at the moment to protect himself. You didn't lash out in anger but exercised the best adaptive mode at the time which was to cope the best that you could. That young child was overpowered by a large adult and did what he could. When this is allowed to occur on a consistent basis the child will not be given the chance to know his own power and strength but instead will go through life feeling helpless. Your job now becomes one of setting and keeping boundaries. Mindfulness training will be your guide. Inserting an element of play will make your job easier.

We each have to respect our own adaptive modes that were utilized in the past. Recognizing these behaviors and the motivations behind them allows you to come to a place where we are able to acknowledge and accept your past actions whether viewed as appropriate or inappropriate. In the process of readjustment you can be thankful for what you have done for yourself in the past and move on. As the old behavior is released, express self gratitude and allow new adaptive behaviors to surface.

In the repeating act of acceptance it is necessary to tell yourself that things are ok just the way they are. Acknowledge your pain and hurt to bring final healing. Acceptance is the ingredient that magically transforms pain into compassion. It is not bad or wrong to experience anger as long as you learn how to use it to your advantage. Anger is a powerful emotion that can be used to achieve goals where otherwise you would just mull along treading water. It is the anger that you are unaware of that can hurt you, slow you down, and make you feel chronically fatigued. Acknowledged anger can be transformed into compassion and action. What will it take to soften and see this and get over your anger? Loving kindness meditation can fill this void.

If you continue to go through life in a stimulus-response mode it is difficult to receive any real insight. Past issues that generated anger will continue to do so. It will take awareness of internal responses to change these angry reactions. Acceptance of anger and limitations will help you become your own friend. People treat you only as well as you treat yourself. Loving yourself becomes a process as well as the ultimate goal.

Even though you may not have felt accepted during childhood now as an adult you can work on self-acceptance. Stop being your own worst critic. Things that we easily excuse in others we hold ourselves responsible for and thus pay the price of self-abuse. What does it take to develop a healthy self-loving? As a child I enjoyed ice cream sandwiches and still enjoy them. The little seven-year-old in my heart smiles when I go for that occasional, after dinner ice cream. From the first thought of the ice cream, to the trip to the freezer, to removing the wrapper, to the first and final bite, there is a feeling of comfort and peace. That feeling lasts long after licking the chocolate from my fingers. It makes my mouth water just to think about it. What things in the past have brought you simple pleasure? Dwell on this question and do what you can to reignite a few of these simple joys.

The same holds true for anger. Just the thought of a troublesome encounter can get the juices flowing and lead to anger. Retelling an anger-provoking event from the past can do the same. There was a day when I would flare up after coming home to find the kitchen sink faucet turned toward the left-hand sink. We have double porcelain sinks that have a movable faucet. It took me six years to figure out why such an insignificant thing would make me angry. While growing up we also had double sinks in our kitchen. The difference back then was that the washing machine was adjacent to the sink and the drain hose from the washing machine hung over into the left hand sink. As the drain screen collected lint and threads there would be an occasional disastrous overflow of dirty laundry water onto the kitchen floor.

To my then untrained mind the faucet of today did not belong over the left side sink since that was the laundry drain side. Only when I recalled that connection was I able to let go and free myself of the aggravation I felt any time I saw the faucet on the "wrong" side. It was never a happy time when the washing machine overflowed and I relived that event every time the facet was to the left even though thirty years had transpired since that experience.

All of the old frustration, anger, and emotional charge was renewed with that vision even though it had occurred so many years ago. I had no awareness of what provoked my anger. Now my washing machine and dryer are far from my kitchen sink but our emotional layer does not forget anything. That faucet posed a danger to my psyche and I was angry because I knew what would happen if that sink overflowed. Memory told me that the left-hand sink was reserved for the dirty laundry water and not for dishes. Any other way would lead to pain as it did one Saturday afternoon when my father in his frustration over the overflow simply threw the evening salad up toward the ceiling leaving it oil marked. I was left to pick up the broken pieces of the bowl.

It took a long time to figure that one out. I was eventually able to bring it to consciousness by realizing that even though I have a wonderful home, in my mind I was still living at 11 North Barnes Street, Waterbury, Connecticut 06704. I needed to accept the fact that I grew up in poverty and acknowledge to myself that by working very hard and making many sacrifices I now live in a very comfortable home. Instead of holding on to my anger over our poverty and our cramped conditions I needed to accept the conditions of the past. Such unwrapping does not come easy, but it is possible. By accepting my past experience I can now walk into my kitchen and not be bothered by the position of the faucet. It is almost hilarious but how many of us go through life allowing little things to rub us the wrong way not knowing why?

As we have been discussing, we need to question and seek the roots of our beliefs. The sink faucet was given so much power because of an inability to deal with a painful experience in real time. As children we lack knowledge and insight into the reasons for the difficulties of others so we unknowingly take the blame for what happens. We remain affected by such events until we can, if ever, many years later, emotionally go back and see the truth in the situation.

What would lead a man to such levels of frustration that he would fling his family's dinner up into the sky? In my father's case he was raising his four children with the help of his mother-in-law because his wife was in and out of psychiatric hospitals. He worked a full time job in a sweat shop and brought home eighty-five dollars a week. With this meager salary he had to pay the rent, buy groceries, put gas in the car and cover repairs. He also had to buy clothes for us, and on Saturday nights put some meat on the table. We learned to deal with frustration in the same ineffective way. It became our job to realize where his beliefs originated and do what we could to restructure them. It has not been easy but with such insights I can slowly get closer to a place where acceptance of my father grows daily. You can do this also.

It will take daily effort and there will be good days and bad days. To resist what is happening at a particular time is to invite suffering into one's life, but to accept what is happening in the moment allows you to avoid getting emotionally entangled. When this becomes evident you are able to make the conscious decision to just allow what is happening to happen and not waste all of your energy on trying to change the reality of the situation.

Pain is a messenger and it is telling you where to focus. It is showing you where you are holding on and not letting life in. It is yelling and telling you to make more space. Instead of moving away from pain and giving in to fear, you can choose to appreciate the pain. Pain is meant to tell you about the way you view life and your existence. The way to ease pain is to listen to it, label it, and become familiar with it. Instead of turning your back on pain, you can face it and learn to appreciate it for what it is. It can be viewed as a necessary and positive experience. Let pain become a teacher by listening to it and momentarily withholding anger and see what comes up. What visions come to mind when you look directly at your pain?

Unpleasant memories will surface as they have been repressed for years. Much of your memory is clouded in interpretations tagged to events viewed subjectively through the eyes of a child. Through introspection you will see that the emotional trauma of years ago is viewed differently through the eyes of a mature adult. By stilling the mind you embrace your pain. If you can commit to not running from what typically frightens you, then you make inroads into awareness. By discovering what makes you tick you find your buttons and neutralize them.

We hold on in so many places and we have held on for so long that the grasping seems natural to us. When we look without judgment at the areas where we are holding on to, a conscious decision to let go can be made. This is a process and everything will not be released in one sitting. From day to day you will notice small internal changes that will translate into external change and overall relaxation. The more relaxed you remain the less tired you find yourself at the end of the day. The more relaxed you are at night the better you are going to sleep.

When there is an inability to work out your issues during the day you will bring them to bed with you and work all night in your dreams. The following morning you awaken feeling more fatigued than when you went to bed. This is one reason why it is necessary to work with your breath during stressful times. The breath acts like a hot knife gliding through butter even on the tightest muscles in our bodies. It takes practice and persistence but you can make it happen. You can localize tension by practicing awareness and release it at will using your breath as a guide. This leads to greater peace and joy as you identify how your thinking affects your feelings.

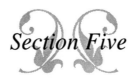

Section Five

OPENING THE HEART

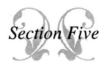

Section Five

OPENING THE HEART

Introduction

*I*t is true today just as it was in the seventeenth century when the
English author John Donne penned the immortal words, "No man is an
island." [1] Everyone is connected and relies on the help of others. This is
especially so when you find yourself in the throes of suffering. Choosing to
remain alone in such a state leaves you bitter, hardened, frozen, and angry.
With the loss of forward motion your creative powers come to a halt and life
no longer seems worth living. In bringing yourself back to a state of a pain-
free existence you will need to renew your trust in your fellow man. Such a
journey is taken one step at a time and is not without its detours and road-
blocks. Your job will be to get to your destination the smoothest way possible utilizing all of the outside help you can surround yourself with.

In order to trust again it is necessary to soften your heart. The pain, frustration, and anger that you have known and that has become your ally needs
to be transformed into forgiveness and acceptance. If you could have
achieved this end to date then you would have. Part of the process in moving
forward is admitting to yourself that you don't know all of the answers and
that it is time to look to others for new perspectives.

The mask that you wear has been for your benefit only. Those around you can easily see through it when they stop and think about it. Think of the energy and will that it takes and how it consumes you just trying to continue living with that mask on. Begin to soften your heart and realize that you are pure and good intrinsically and have no need to hide anything from others or yourself.

One of the most effective ways of helping yourself is to reach out and help others. When you remove yourself from your self-centeredness for more than a few minutes at a time you can easily see that there are others who suffer just as much and even more than you do. Once this becomes clear to you and your self-acceptance begins to blossom you will naturally want to reach out and serve those in need. As you accept the fact that you also have needs that have to be met and move mindfully in the direction of meeting them you will feel more alive than you ever have. You will find that you can appreciate everything that has ever happened to you, good and bad.

In the following final chapters we will be discussing effective, non-threatening ways for expressing your needs to those in your circles. In addition the skills and practice of fostering and maintaining healthy relationships and support systems during times of transition will be presented. We will conclude with an exploration of personal intention and how that fits in with a life of service to others.

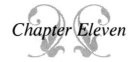

Chapter Eleven

Looking to Others

*W*e think we are alone but we are not. Five billion people live on our earth sharing the same space and air. Feeling singled out and isolated, the alienation surrounding our attitude toward our problems leaves us in irons, stranded hundreds of miles from the peace, rest, companionship, and community that we need. The human connections that provide healing balm are obviously lacking and we imagine that nobody knows the trouble we've seen. Thus we feel alone and perpetuate the hard held belief that no one understands us. "They" just don't know what we have to go through and put up with every day. We are disconnected from others and are unaware that the roots of this disconnect are our attitudes and beliefs concerning ubiquitous problems.

A strong sense of self-induced isolation exists because we delude ourselves about the reality of our lives. It is as if we have a need to star in the lead role of a drama and that drama just so happens to be our life. In the middle of this loneliness our minds concoct all sorts of hindering and self-limiting stories. It is as if we are afraid of our own boredom. Chogyam Trungpa tells us in his book, *The Myth of Freedom and the Way of Meditation*,[1] that in order to begin to get insight into our own stories we need to get to a place where we can appreciate boredom. In meditation we need to drop any concept of reward. The attitude we take should be one of just sitting with ourselves watching the breath without any intention of control. Any thought of having a goal negates the meaning of mindfulness. In his words we need to get rid of our credentials and part of our credentials is our identification with sickness and or pain.

How many of us are motivated by what others think of us, depending on the approval of others to feel truly good about ourselves? In this mindset we find ourselves looking to others with the wrong motivation. Many individuals hide behind higher degrees and titles depending on the credentials and hard work that it took to earn these titles. Living from this prospective has you using others in the sense that they are there for you to impress. Even if you do not have a higher degree, do you use the fact that you are the breadwinner as a way of expecting special treatment and or respect at home? Do you use your intimate connection with your pain as a way of getting the attention you seek and need?

It is not necessary or advisable to tell everyone all of your intimate secrets but it is healthy to have one or two individuals with whom you can speak from the heart and not worry about repercussions. Afraid to bear our souls to others we think that what we tell someone in confidence may someday be used against us when we least expect it. Now we are told that in order to make progress in a mindfulness practice we have to drop our credentials. You may be a mom or a dad, a doctor or a lawyer, a carpenter or a mason, but underneath the role you are made of the same flesh and blood as everyone who has ever walked this earth. It is hard to admit to our own faulty thinking but until we do so we find we are living our own prescription for suffering.

We have more in common than we care to admit especially in the arena of suffering. Our intrinsic worth has been diluted by socialization but it can be rekindled by spending meditative time with yourself and moving your new found wisdom into action through daily acts of courage. Such acts may be sitting with an ailing parent, stopping at the grocery store for a disabled neighbor, or shoveling snow from an elderly neighbor's door. I call these acts of courage because in order to do these things you have to momentarily put someone else first, before yourself. These small favors move you away from the vice of self-centeredness and allow you to express the virtue of generosity. These small acts of kindness will bring you closer to others, get you out of the seeking mode, and offer you the opportunity of giving of yourself. Our worth goes deeper than our titles. What is it about Western society that tells us that we have to make something of ourselves and strive and work hard to prove our worth? Status anxiety is just an idea. It doesn't mean that we have to live up to it. As you begin to assist others in simple tasks you will find that their sincere "Thank you," is enough to melt your heart and help you to feel wanted and needed. This is all that any one of us wants.

There is another way to look to others. We can begin practicing compassion and begin to relate to others the way Eugen Herrigel describes in *The Method of Zen*. We can make it a practice to relate to each other on a "solar plex to solar plex level." He describes the art of compassion by telling how a Zen priest helps a sufferer endure his suffering in the right way. The goal is not to relieve the suffering or to question why the suffering was brought on in the first place but "salvation lies in giving full assent to his fate, serenely accepting what is laid upon him without asking why he should be singled out for so much suffering." Detachment occurs and this detachment is what leads to healing. The healing process unfolds as one becomes more sensitive to the suffering of others.[2] Can you begin to open you eyes to the suffering of others and not draw back in fear?

The sympathy that I talked about in Chapter Two while discussing the death of the young man who left behind his wife of thirteen years, a six-year-old daughter, and three-year-old son is according to Herrigel a sentimental sympathy. This kind of sympathy is easily aroused and quickly dissipated. The reason for this he believes is because the sympathy is not selfless enough. Fellow suffering on the other hand is the mark of true compassion. In selflessly sharing another's suffering one can experience healing.

It is difficult to truly share another's suffering. It is draining and makes us prone to tears. Sensitivity is not something that is fostered in young Americans. Many times I have heard a parent tell a young child not to cry even when they are hurt. The child is told to be tough and that big kids don't cry. Even worse the child may be admonished and be told not to be a sissy. In our house, Treva especially makes it a priority to let the guys feel what they are feeling. The teaching here is that it is OK to feel sad. It is Ok to cry if you're tired. It is Ok to struggle, though I like to step in when the frustration level gets to a point where one of the guys begins to come down on himself. We as parents are here to help our children but we are also assigned the task of helping them become independent and responsible adults.

We all need to be more acutely aware of our own responsibilities. An interesting exercise is to live a day with the thought that we no longer have the capacity to blame anyone for our predicaments. Our internal response in this imagined day could be that no matter what uncomfortable feelings arise, the predominant reason we feel so bad is because of an attitude we have had in the past that we refuse to let go of. In this courageous exercise we are to accept the concept that everything that happens to us is an opportunity for healing. At some level, many times at a subconscious level, because of the need to maintain defense mechanisms, we desired all of the results that came to us, knowing that working through these problems will bring wholeness. No one else had anything to do with it and there is no one to blame, not even ourselves. What changes would we make in our thinking and attitudes if we lived like this and truly knew the power of our own thoughts and words?

We can look to others to lessen the blow when it comes to how hard we are on ourselves. Many times others are more forgiving and understanding than we are when we make mistakes. We make mistakes and say things we don't really mean especially when we are tired. We have our own ideas about a situation and come down hard on ourselves coloring the rest of the day in gloom at our lack of sensitivity. A spouse or friend may come along and point out the great degree the stress we have been under, or how we haven't had adequate sleep because of other demands. They help us lighten our load. Others can help heal our wounds and most of the time they don't even know they are doing it. Be open to this.

Most people will go out of their way to help others. Look to others to see how they are suffering and how you might begin to compassionately share in that suffering instead of looking for what they can do for you. This can be done effectively, with a degree of detachment, as long as it is approached in a mindful way. Being aware of what we are doing in trying to share in another's suffering brings us across an imaginary line into the circle of the other's life. We begin to share being, connected and moving to the same vibrations. Understanding begins to unfold and greater trust results. In trusting others we make strides in trusting life and our own path widens.

Begin to ask yourself, how can what another individual experiences help me unfold and see my place in the world? Where do I fit in the scheme of things and what do I do best that reaches out to others? Begin to look to others as recipients of your good thoughts and actions. Start sharing your talents instead of hiding your light under a bushel.Looking to others may not be as easy as it seems. We are all led to believe that we have to be strong and not show any weakness. It is like wearing a mask, putting on a front all of the time, and projecting the image that we are self-sufficient; otherwise we are viewed as needy. It is appropriate to be needy when the need is real. Complaining comes across as whining when others see that you possess the ability to take care of yourself but for whatever reason you choose not to. They wonder why you do not take the necessary steps to get your needs met since you have what you need to do so. In their eyes your "suffering" pales in comparison to theirs. You end up losing respect and not being heard.

When you need attention from others, look to those who have demonstrated a caring attitude in the past. When you come with this intention at the forefront of your thoughts you begin to search for results even before you actually ask for help. You have taken the steps to open your heart and listen within to helpful and caring attitudes that you have heard expressed in the past. You know these attitudes work, you remember, and open up more fully, grateful for the caring thoughts of others. You are not alone and do not have to depend totally on yourself. Instead of feeling angry, confused, and lost, you feel grateful.

Many marriages go on with both parties unhappy continuing in roles where one player is lazy and the other takes it on themselves to get everything done. Some in their marriages are fortunate to have a strong partner. This partner strives to remain aware of their partner's needs and when necessary takes charge to get their partner motivated to make tough changes. In an optimal marriage the volley goes back and forth and it is not always the same partner who takes the lead. Everyone cycles having periods of effectiveness when everything they try or do turns out right. On the down side of the cycle it seems like all efforts are stalled and nothing gets done. It may even feel like your taking steps backwards. This is just the way life works. When you work to increase your awareness of yourself you are able to recognize these cycles in yourself and others. It takes trust to allow another to take the initiative especially when you may be the one who is accustomed to running the show. It doesn't make you any less of a person to allow yourself to accept help. This is especially so when you have been suffering from chronic pain no matter what the cause.

In looking to others there are numerous ways to see what we can do to help. In our efforts we find that we are the one's who actually benefit. Teaching yoga to patients, family members, and staff has become a gift of giving for me. The turn out is variable, but if there are three people participating or ten people I always find that I learn more about my own yoga practice by instructing others. Watching to see who might be holding their breath with a pose, or who is struggling, contorting their facial muscles when they should be completely relaxed, released, and composed, allows and opportunity for connection. When someone is working too hard at a pose suggestions are made that allow for the release of unnecessary effort. Much of the instruction is about opening enough to allow the participants to question themselves about why they believe they need to hold on to what they are holding on to. As trust builds, comfort and ease replace trying.

We all have a tendency to compare ourselves to those around us. To a degree this is reasonable in that it gives us something to work toward. When we make comparisons with a critical eye we are headed for trouble. This can take us to a place where nothing is ever satisfying and the comparing can go on the rest of your life unless you wake up and stop it yourself. In looking to others and seeing what they have it is easier on yourself to be happy for them than to harbor jealousy. Their manifestations can be viewed as evidence that it can also happen for you. Instead of feeling angry that your neighbor has no concept of the pain that you are experiencing, and that life for them appears perfect on the surface, appreciate the fact that this person is able to go through life without significant pain. It simply means that such a way of life is there for you also. You may need to do a great deal of reparative work to get there, but proceeding along these lines is so much better than continuing on with your current pain path.

It takes time to undo what stress has done to a body over years. Revelations concerning what has to be undone come slowly and they are painful both, mentally and physically. We are all beginners. Do your best and be honest with yourself. Allow yourself the gift of other's experience and go to those who you believe can offer assistance. They will give you the gift of showing you your own progress. Through the compassion of others you will gain a sense of hope that your pain might continue to improve to the point that someday it will not consume you. Continuing to look at your practice as a process allows you to be where you are with less concern over comparisons.

Become your own teacher. Ask others for help when you need it but then take what they give you and apply that information to your own life. Only you know what will work best for you so use the ideas and experience of others to get jump-started onto a new track. Even thirty minutes a day intentionally placing your thoughts and hopes toward what you want to see manifest in your life will show you that even in the worst of circumstances there will be positive change. You may not make great strides but any change away from the ordinary can be enough to carry you through your toughest times and challenges.

All of your past inertia has left you with tight tendons, ligament, muscles, and fascia. Lacking any extra energy an exercise program is the last thing you would want to undertake, but now is the time to think about a friend or acquaintance who might be suffering in the same way that you are and invite them to start a regular walking program with you. If you have a local YMCA it would be a great idea to use the pool and walk laps together three times a week. Water has its own healing powers and even has the potential to spark your creative imaginings.

It is time to finally make the decision to take care of you. In the process you will give others the chance to feel useful as you ask for their assistance. As you begin to break through old rigid thinking everything looks new. A fluid body makes for a fluid mind and this new sense of ease will be expressed in everything that you do. Tight thinking is all around us. As you loosen up you will begin to notice how others hold themselves and how they move and interact with others. Your new found ease with your own condition will make it easier for you to relate to others who are where you have been. This places you in a position to help them and the more you are able to assist others the more appreciation you will experience for your own situation.

As you learn what it takes to loosen tight hamstrings and relive low back pain you will be more able to convey this information to others who have noticed the new spring in your step. You will be able to see who and who has not made the intention to take care of themselves. You can see someone's twisted neck and ask what is it that they are so uptight about? Why is it that they feel they cannot trust to receive healing? What is it that they are telling themselves that puts them in such a painful position and what makes them want to hold on to such beliefs? There are many things that we do to ourselves that we are unaware of. In our interactions with others, they unknowingly show us where we can make changes in our beliefs, but we need to be mindful that these demonstrations are available with each interpersonal interaction.

As Chogyam Trunpa says we need to get to the place where we realize that everything around us reflects our state of inner being. Everything around us is meant to be a road map to greater living. In looking to others we melt the self- induced isolation that we feel and allow ourselves to dance with others. In that dance we find our true place and value. Others will want to attempt what you have done in an effort to induce positive change in their lives. The more confidence you experience the more willing you will be to put yourself out there for others. In looking to others we can see who and who does not take care of themselves then make the conscious decision to be there for them as others have been there for us.

Chapter Twelve

The Path to Health is Paved with Intention

*L*essons we learn from the movies tell us to move forward and never look back no matter what. In real life in order to move forward it is sometimes necessary to look back to the past to see how we arrived just where we are. This is an intentional process in which we work to unlock ourselves from frozen emotions. These emotions were the result of personal trauma, long buried by defense mechanisms that were meant to protect us from their hurtful effects. Until we know how we arrived it will be difficult to go exactly where we want to go. Living in the past or longing for the good old days is not what I am talking about. Instead, reviewing past events with all of their associated feelings and emotions, not just good and bad, but those you view as indifferent is encouraged.

Reviewing and analyzing your reactions to significant events in your life is a useful habit that will help to fine-tune your new course of action. In playing back memories and reviewing painful events you are able to loosen the paralyzing grip they possess over you. Painful events get locked into memory banks and color every thought and action that you experience. Over time there develops the loss of the capacity and know-how of getting around the cement wall that has been built between the conscious and unconscious selves. Muscles have memory and once locked in it takes extraordinary measures, lead by an intentional desire to unlock the messages hidden in these muscles.

The natural tendency is to avoid painful memories. We expend incredible amounts of energy keeping the past at bay, keeping it where we think it cannot hurt us. Because we continue to function at a reasonable level we allow the past to maintain its grip on us. The price is fatigue and a decreased sense of being truly alive. If our past was as simple as a time line in history it might be easier to unravel past problems. Instead the past has side roads, alleys, cul-de-sacs, mountainous curves, peaks, and valleys. There are tunnels and crevasses, dirt roads, and cow paths. The paths are not straight and orderly and emotions and feelings are interwoven and enmeshed. Some are stuck together with the strongest of epoxies and the way to dissolve these glues will take many avenues, many attempts, and a great deal of assistance from others. Most of all it will take your intent.

Your intention is the fuel that will get you started on this path and it will also be the source of energy that will allow you to persist in moving toward your goal of complete health even when things begin to look darker. We can have multiple feelings over the same situation. The bittersweet of life that makes a good movie good is the same bittersweet that makes a life meaningful, colorful, and lived. We all have fond memories of the past. Unfortunately, because of the stresses of our days, even the heartwarming and mind soothing memories are buried deep. Intentionally taking time to daydream about the past or about the future is time well spent. This can be done with mindfulness and is not done in a daze or without thought. It can be a time to regenerate our much depleted batteries.

By taking the time and doing the work to unravel the past you come to a place where you experience inner peace in spite of what is going on around you. You now have the ability to take a stand and not feel mauled over when someone else comes at you with their stuff. Their harmful thoughts, actions, and emotions need not do you any harm as you realize that you own your own power and have not given anyone else the ability to push your buttons. This allows you to act and not react to any situation. In an attempt to relieve their own suffering others can unintentionally try to make their suffering part of your problem. By working at untying the past you come to know yourself and develop greater definition of your boundaries. A warning flag automatically rises when someone tries to cross the line and dump their stuff on you. With the knowledge of your past you are able to stop them in their tracks and gently allow them to accept their own shortcomings. You are able to get out of the way of others' expectations and let them feel what they are feeling without any associated guilt.

Our minds have ingrained patterns that have developed over thousands and thousands of past events. Chemical and hormonal events occur to make us what we are. This occurs faster than we could ever imagine. We have learned how to respond to others from the sacred place within but also from family influences and expectations. Our ideas of who we are may not be in tune with what and who others think we are. In working to unravel the past, it is our own voice we are trying to hear more clearly. So much of what goes on within is on the unconscious level. With work, effort and intention, you can bring more of these hidden aspects of your being to the surface.

Our children go to Montessori. There is a new directress there who has mentioned to Treva that she can really tell that we talk and listen to our boys by the way they express themselves and how they process information. Unfortunately many parents do not listen to their children. The children go unheard and are spoken to as if they were not human.

Many children are told what to do and how to act and feel by well-meaning parents, but then they go through the rest of their lives unable to think and problem solve effectively on their own. This is very sad. How we get over this type of behavior is by going back to the days when this was what we were hearing. Emotionally reliving these events and playing them out in your mind, you can make new assessments from your higher self. Decisions can be made from the point of view of the best possible outcome for you. You always want to be thinking what the right thing to do in this moment is best for you.

In reliving and unraveling the past it is necessary that we become observers. It is our choice to confront painful internal images just as it is our choice to run from them by washing the dishes, mopping the floor, mowing the lawn, or even lashing out at a loved one because the images cause us irritability. It is necessary to sit with the image and be in a position of unresponsiveness to the image. In the place of non-responsiveness you allow yourself to experience exactly why you are holding on to that image. For me most of my holding on occurs in my right mandibular or jaw region. This causes right neck and facial pain as well as a chronic pulling sensation of the upper part of the chest because of tension within the scalene muscles.

We have to be able to cry with ourselves and for ourselves, unashamed of our tears. The greatest healing comes when you embrace your tears and find yourself in the center of your personal sorrow. I am not saying that we need to feel sorry for ourselves, but we need to identify and acknowledge our sorrow and loneliness.

By going back in the mind, in a safe manner, without excitement or fear, you allow yourself to retouch the trauma of the past. Like still water, your mind will not run from the scenes of past hurts. Instead your heart will be drawn toward the pain and healing will occur. The relief of past sorrow is the work of the heart but first you must allow the heart to soften. There has to be room and allowance for the heart to open so that it can feel, touch, and know the hurt. Through this identification with the heart you are getting out of the way of your body's own intelligence to heal itself. By holding on to the attitude that you are too busy to slow down and practice you allow your suffering to continue on its never ending cycle.

Where are you going that makes you believe that you can't take time for yourself? You are what your past has made you by choice and it will continue on unless you do something about it. Your own issues bother you. The issues of others bother you also and everyone puts off doing anything about it by distraction. Through the art of mindfulness we will eventually see all of the connections in our lives. Some say that we will even be able to experience past lives. Our being is really a mystery and it will probably remain a mystery for a long, long, time, but there is nothing to stop us from living this mystery and being a part of it. There is no reason why anyone has to be the victim of fate or circumstances.

To be what we want to be we first must discover who we are. We will never be able to reclaim the past but we can go back into the past and use the lessons to give us greater presence now. It takes a degree of self- leadership and a strong willingness to rebuild from the past. In the process we can accept what we are now but we can also know that there is much more to us below the surface. By digging into past experience we extract gems of insight and knowledge that had previously been allowed to escape our consciousness. We are creatures of conditioning. Look at what Pavlov has shown us, but this doesn't mean that we are powerless over our circumstances.

The past need not be associated with a negative connotation. As I recall my junior high school days playing strawberry in gym class, I am able to rekindle the competitive spirit I drew upon at the age of fifteen. Over the past many years I had lost that competitive edge and began to feel that I needed to compete against no one except myself. This belief kept me away from anything competitive. I was so self-conscious that when I would attempt anything of a competitive nature my self-consciousness would hinder any type of high performance. In an effort to avoid more hurt to my ego I stopped competing. In doing so I believe that I lost out on a great deal of high energy, self-renewing, life affirming actions. Looking back to those high school days I can tell myself that yes I was able to participate and I was able to participate well. I walked away with the pulse of life beating in my veins.

We all have had high points in our life. It helps to reflect on our winnings in the past even if they were small winnings. Such contemplation benefits us especially when we are feeling down. We are made up of so many parts that to avoid the winners within or the warriors within we do ourselves a disservice.

Family members are an excellent source of information when it comes to the actual facts of our past. This past Thanksgiving my Aunt Mary and sister Mary were here to visit. Before they arrived I had the intention of talking with my aunt to ask her specific questions about my mother. I wanted to know what she was like before she married my father. With legal pad and pen I began asking my questions and jotting down notes. Even though I heard the answers from my aunt I wanted to write down what was said, as I know I will want to go back to the answers to review later. We all process information and come up with our own ideas about what was said. Time and serious thought allow for greater insight than just making a judgment at the moment something is heard. I know what we had discussed will come up spontaneously in my morning meditation. From this point my mind will take me where it needs to and my job is to just follow the thoughts and see what comes up. I hope to see my mother and her life in a new light.

One story was about summer Saturday trips to the beach. My mother and her girlfriend Mary, are you getting the picture of our nationality with all of the Mary's, would take my aunt with them to Ocean Beach by bus. They would pack a lunch and walk to the bus station on the Green, in downtown Waterbury. After getting on the bus it was a long ride to Bridgeport as this was long before route eight was built. They would spend the day on the beach. My aunt enlightened me when she mentioned that my mother and her friend would talk to the boys. She stressed that they talked to the boys a lot. It seems that she would know because she was much younger and could not go off on her own but had to hang out with her sister and friend.

This new mental picture of my mother shows me another side of her, which in the past I was never aware of. I simply recall a mom who I would make cookies with, who worked only for a short time out of the house when I was young, and who while I was still young ended up going in and out of hospitals then ended up living in a nursing home. The memories that I have are of a withdrawn, quiet, and depressed woman. To know that she had a life and lived with some spark in the past will help me reframe her image and my own. Right now I do not know how all of this new information is going to be of help but I do know that it will help unfold some of the mysteries that are within.

Looking to the past for insight will help unravel the hidden questions we all have. To move into the past momentarily from a gentle, quiet place within will bring waves of healing to our shore.

To feel as a child does and be able to play brings new vigor to your life. As you open to a mindset that seeks joy it gets easier to do the things that make you happy. Devoid of the attitude of play, fatigue shackles you. You gain energy when you look for ways to make your work more playful. The work I am referring to is not only your vocation but also the inner work you will be doing to bring your life into balance. It is all right to be serious but even in these moments there can be room for lightness and play without necessarily joking around. Reading the Buddhist texts we find that we are all living in a dream. We pass our time unaware of this and continue to live out our stories, complete with illusions, delusions, doubts, and fears. It is our mission to awaken from that dream. Play is the vehicle that allows us to accomplish this goal by reducing our suffering and dropping us into the present moment.

I used to believe that being innocent was a sign of weakness or immaturity. Now I see innocence as a state of openness that has the capacity to usher change in our lives. We diminish our effectiveness by holding on to ideas and thus get out of synch with what is before us in this moment. Innocence makes us approachable. Others will sense this imperturbable attitude and know that we are available to them in their time of need. In this state of mind, questions and clarification flow easily without making the questioner feel inferior or lacking. You must view yourself as a questioner also and take it easy on yourself so that you can hear the answers to your own life transforming questions.

You are both a member and the captain of your own team. The fostering of team spirit allows all aspects of your personality to get involved in seeking the answers that you need. You will feel good about this new approach to problem solving and as you continue on in a playful mindset, the drudgery of life is forgotten and the lighter sides of things are allowed center stage. More positive attitudes prevail in such an environment.

Pure play is timeless. It is being in action. Play allows for acceptance of the self in the moment and allows us to drop time constraints and the nagging sense of self. A child picks up a stick, swings it in the air and is transferred to a world of imagination and wonder. The shine on his face and the glazed wonder in the eyes tells us that he is in a holy place. That stick has become a toy. The imagination is in high gear and soars spontaneously. No one is forcing the child to play. The desire has arisen without prompting. The energy could have come from the ground or the sky. It is there and the child utilizes it without question. No goal is evident but the child feels the movement of his arm as he swings. As he strikes an object with his stick his entire being is one with the impact, then the vibration. These sensations are experienced first in his fingers and hands, then his arms, and eventually dissipate throughout his entire being.

As reviewed in *The Childhood Roots of Adult Happiness* by Edward M. Hallowell, M.D., play is one of the needs of children.[1] He hopes, as I do, that play will go on though-out life. His concern with society today is the current parental need for seeing children lead enriched lives. Treva and I are as guilty as the next set of parents as we have John Trey going from school, to bells at church, to tennis lesson, to piano lessons, all on a Thursday afternoon. On Saturdays, now that soccer season is over, there is basketball at the YMCA. We console ourselves by rationalizing that we did not force John Trey to take piano lessons. If we had our way we would have wanted him to start lessons at the age of three, like the rest of the child prodigies in the world. Instead we waited until he asked us about it. We gave him the option of holding off with basketball this season but he chose to participate.

The positive in all of these activities is that it gives me a chance to interact with John Trey as he practices at home. Like many of our neighbors we have a portable basketball goal. At fifty inches tall he still has a good distance to throw the ball to score but his free throws are getting more accurate. He has not yet practiced his lay ups but they too will come with time. Not to leave Joel out of it, I will pick him up while he has the basketball clenched to his chest. This is no easy task, as he now weighs thirty-six pounds. At hoop height he will drop the ball into the net and score. His face lights up knowing that he too can get two points.

Over the Thanksgiving holiday I spent some time getting a talk together to present to the Norfolk Oncology Nursing Society. While I spent my time in the study, Treva and the guys were decorating the outside bushes with Christmas lights. As the afternoon passed and the sun began to fall into the horizon, a small voice in my head told me to go outside and play with my boys. The next day I would be back at work and they would be back at school. So as Treva and her cousin continued stringing the lights, Joel, John Trey and I ran around the front yard. Our play eventually led us to the basketball hoop. Joel wanted me to pick him up so that he could score. We have one of those Fisher-Price plastic basketball hoops, but he was to have nothing of that while I was around to pick him up. I did what I could to encourage him to play with the little hoop but he kept on that he wanted me to pick him up to the big basket. Even at the small hoop he doesn't have the arm strength to make a basket on his own. In a flash there is a vision of Joel standing on a platform to make his shots. The recycling container, a very hard rectangular plastic box, places him six inches from the hoop. When John Trey saw this he wanted to join us so he took the ball and started doing slam-dunks into the small basket. John Trey would do a slam-dunk then I would get the rebound and hand off to Joel who would slide the ball through the hoop for two points. I then had John Trey move ten to fifteen feet away, let Joel make his shot, get the rebound and pass to John Trey who would grab the ball, dribble to the hoop and score with a nice lay-up shot. I threw in the sound effects and we were transported to a championship game in Madison Square Garden playing the game of our lives. Everyone was happy. John Trey did his lay-ups, Joel got to score and I got to experience tremendous joy with my boys. Our imaginations were going wild and in the process of play the boys were able to work on the mastery of the game, practice their motor skills, and develop greater hand-eye coordination. They were able to accomplish all of this without the associated frustrations they usually experience when they miss a shot. If a shot was missed it was not a big deal as the action was moving so fast there was no time to get bogged down.

It's ok to become frustrated but there are degrees of frustration that can manifest in all of us that leave us paralyzed. As Hallowell says, "Play teaches the ability to tolerate frustration and it teaches the all-important ability to fail." [2] Joel seems to get very frustrated with even one miss. I have found the best thing to do at his age is to let him make all of the shots by putting him in a position where he cannot miss. John Trey, being older, fully understands that he will not make all of his shots and if he hits even fifty percent he considers that a success.

In writing about play I find that it is difficult to find the right place for play in everyday life. All of the effort that we expend in meeting the demands of the day takes away much of our precious energy. The distractions over the needs of others seem to drain the very life out of us. Our resistance to meeting our own needs, and those of others, is what actually wears us down. It is our reluctance to just allow things to happen as they were meant to happen that makes us fight the present moment. We can find peace by allowing ourselves to surrender to whatever comes up. It may be that in such moments, no matter what the gravity of the situation, if we are able to let life in then life itself will show us how to play. Giving in but not giving up is the key.

We have to keep our eyes and our senses open to the vibration of the moment. In reading more about meditation and breathing I have discovered that the simple act of taking a breath can be joyful and pleasurable in itself. This can be reason enough to be in the moment and be happy that we are alive.

By maintaining an attitude of playfulness even in serious work we no longer become victims to the moods and constraints of others. We all can do more than one thing at once. In today's society it is in vogue to multitask, so why not do so to our own advantage? You can do your serious work and on the inside where everything really counts you can remain playful. For myself at work while I am listening to a patient's concerns I am able to also pay attention to my breathing and in the process watch my own reactions to what I am hearing. As another example at work, when I find myself getting run down by the sheer number of patients that I see in a day, I find that the more I resist what I am called to do the greater my suffering. When I make a conscious decision to keep going without my own editorial input I seem to get into a flow state and my worst fears do not materialize.

During the course of the day I also listen to the breath sounds and the heart sounds of my patients. This is an excellent opportunity to pay attention to my own rhythms and get into the moment. These techniques give me more inner space and helps me feel more comfortable in my own skin. In such a frame of mind, activities become timeless, moods are lifted and you do not allow yourself to dwell on the heaviness of life. You become light and those around you soften and are allowed to share in your lightness. It is healthy to give yourself this gift. If you live with this intention on a daily basis, everyone you come in contact with will benefit. This simple choice tells you and the world that you have chosen to take care of yourself. As you become more adept at taking care of yourself you place yourself in a better position to help others do the same for themselves.

Conclusion

COMING FULL CIRCLE

ow that you have come this far you will have discovered that this is only the beginning of your journey. Make allowances so that you move along at your own pace. Remember, we are trying to slow things down enough so the true voice within becomes audible. There will be times when things happen quickly and smoothly, one right after the other, and events will present themselves just as imagined. At other times there will be periods of frustration, anger, and feelings that nothing you do will ever work out. During these times it is acceptable to slow your pace, spend more time in self-restoration, and possibly seek out new avenues of assistance like spiritual or psychological counseling, a second opinion from a medical specialists, a referral to a pain specialist, acupuncture, massage therapy, or a meditation and or yoga retreat.

The information shared in this book is meant to act as a guide in your search for wholeness, health, and fulfillment. There are no easy or quick ways to achieve these goals. It is my hope that you will keep coming back to the chapters that speak to you, and in doing so, discover new insights with each encounter. You have learned how powerful past experience can be in helping you decide a new course of action. The knowledge that past traumatic experiences can be catalytic and transformative has given you a powerful tool. The source of that power was locked up, frozen, and dormant. Now through the practice of daily meditation and a few basic yoga asanas, you have in your possession the keys that will turn up the heat, melt the ice, and get the molecules of imagination and creation moving again.

Getting started by taking a panoramic view of where you are and determining where you want to go gives you your best options. They will present themselves to you when you take things a step at a time. Only you know what is best for you, but even under optimal circumstances some of your choices may at first make you think that you have made a wrong decision. Do not judge your actions or their consequences. As long as your intentions are right your needs will be met. Choose to let go of the pressures of time and performance and allow your mind to drop into each moment as much as you are capable.

You now have the knowledge and resources to rebuild your life one brick at a time. With the realization that the process is in a constant state of flux, your main goal is one of remaining open and adaptable to new feelings and situations. The idea of change will no longer scare you. Instead you will be open to the excitement that a new way of feeling, thinking, acting, and being will bring. Your ability to find new sources of energy has expanded many- fold, and as you systematically disengage from your energy drains, you will learn to divert your precious energy to the creation of the life that you have always wanted. Problems will be viewed as opportunities to exercise your ever expanding creative energies.

We have discussed, in depth, the desire for self-protection and how remaining in such a mind set only keeps your energy locked up. As you drop your shields and open your heart you will at times feel greater pain, but it will be the pain that we all feel. You are not alone. As your compassion grows you will find just how kind and generous you can be not only to others, but also toward your family and yourself. As the process of building trust proceeds you find that your pain is your greatest advisor. If you choose to listen to its message your priorities change. Old, worn out, drag me down beliefs will start to be questioned, and you will start to live.

As awareness expands you find yourself living in the moment more and more. All hell may break loose to the left of you, things may be falling apart to the right of you, but as you practice walking in the middle of it all, you discover that you have become an instrument of positive change. Present in the middle ground, remaining centered, and acting instead of reacting, your actions and words will demonstrate to others that they too can live with an open heart. You will still feel pain, but now you know that you are not your pain, you are not the cause of your pain, and you are strong enough to show others how to work with their pain. Pain has become a tool used for growth and positive change.

You are now fully aware of the power of your breath. As you breathe so will you live. Breathe fully and you will live fully. As you continue to work with the exercises found within *Passion Beyond Pain*, you will appreciate this power more and more. You will navigate your way through depression, cut short the hindering ravages of anxiety, and know that it is wise to ask for help when needed. As you build the courage to question your beliefs, there will be times of heightened anxiety; there will be times when you will not feel in control, and times when you will not know what is going to happen. These are the times that you will be living at your fullest; times that are devoid of self-centeredness and that are full of potential. As you break away from old, self-defeating habits you discover new ways of achieving that which you really need to live fully. You find that you have definite choices at every point and you will be able to avert crisis situations.

You have been introduced to the concept of the ancient *chakra* system. The knowledge gained through examining each of the *chakras* and working with them is not only cumulative but also synergistic. You may play with the ideas for a day or so, get busy doing something else, then find yourself feeling fully grounded and present as you incorporate the principles learned from working with the *chakras*. This may happen as you take care of your garden, wash your car, or confront a difficult person or situation. It is important to state here that the concepts dealt with in working with the *chakras* are in no way associated with any religious beliefs. It is simply a way of viewing our energy centers that has been handed down since ancient times.

Through your readings new insight has surfaced relating to the constant communication that occurs within your body. You now know how to allow the healthy parts of your mind and body to gently speak to and direct those areas that are in need of healing. You have discovered your own inner healer, and have on the tip of your tongue, the words to tell yourself that will allow immediate, though at first temporary, restoration.

You now appreciate the power of optimism and see the destructive nature of catastrophizing and are ready to remain aware of all that you think and speak. Whatever comes your way is viewed as an opportunity to remain present and not simply labeled as good or bad. You are connecting with yourself and thus will have deeper relationships with those you love.

At this time you are beginning to realize that the energy of your anger has a purpose. You have discovered that anger in itself is not to be judged, but is a resource you can call upon to help get you moving in the direction of your choice. This energy can propel you toward your goals. Instead of burning up inside with such intense feelings, you are able to direct the anger, manipulate it, and make friends with it, just as you are able to make friends with all of your previously buried emotions, that in the past only served to leave you frightened.

By listening to the inner voice and encouraging kind communication, you uncover the power that you so feared. You are now in a position to see that fear is only fear, and you will do what you want despite the fear. You have removed the paralyzing power of fear by confronting it and seeing it for what it is: empty thought, once full of power only because you gave into it. This is no longer the case. You are in charge and now walk the middle path in awareness.

As your new life opens up you find yourself in a position to welcome the work ahead. Each time you drop an old belief system that previously made you the victim you feel an incredible sense of relief. The rocks in your pockets have been removed and your steps are lighter. The flames are burning and they are the fuel that separates you from past harmful behaviors. The flames light your way and purify any notions of holding on to guilt or shame. You are happy to feel the heat.

You may begin to see just how much anger you have been holding inside as your dreams become more vivid. You awaken in the morning with a new understanding and are not afraid to share your insights with a confidant. In the past the pain put out the fire, where now the pain is one with the fire and even though there may still be a component of pain present, it is not of the same intensity that in the past left you paralyzed. The heat allows you to look at difficult emotions with the intention of overcoming them. It will not be easy but now you have more energy, greater stamina, and increased confidence to come to the middle and live. The desire to hide and run from your problems will lessen and your determination to be who you are will show you the steps to take to remain on your path.

As you develop greater proficiency in working with your breath you will find yourself less anxious. The places where you would previously hold on to nervous tension will make themselves known. Under your direction they will loosen up as you begin to experience a new found sense of liberation. You find yourself satisfied and thankful for what you have. Grateful for the next breath, you have moved to a higher plane of living.

As you perform the exercises throughout this book your awareness of your internal dialogue and repressed feelings will increase. Your job will be to stick with the work and seek out the help you need when you need it. If the pain intensifies to the point where you are in need of more pain medicine or more muscle relaxers then use them as you need to. Once you reduce the cycle of pain and frustration your need for these medicines will decrease. This is not to say that you may not need them at a later date, but the hope is that the intervals between their uses will lengthen.

Through all of this work hopefully you will have discovered that your fire does not have to burn twenty-four hours a day. It is healthy to take care of yourself and take breaks. Workaholics suffer from a disease just as alcoholics do. The problem is that when one suffers from working in excess, their efforts are rewarded and it is especially difficult to come to center in these cases. It can be accomplished, but it will take more effort and determination. We all have a choice to walk the middle path. Once you make this decision your life and the lives of those around you will be enriched.

Though your readings you will have benefited from a working knowledge of your other "bodies," or the five *koshas*. With time and practice you will develop the ability to enhance your awareness down to a pre-thought level. You will intuitively know what you need to do, when you need to do it, and how to remain in balance. As you build trust in working with your different levels your inner wisdom and respect will show you just how important each individual is in the life of others. Through suffering and living with chronic pain there is much that has been forgotten. Through the use of meditation you will reconnect with the visions once held and become child-like in your approach to all things. You will find joy in things as simple as the wind blowing your hair. These are things that money cannot buy, yet they are the things that you can teach your children. Do so and the world will be the benefactor.

Through the practice of loving kindness meditation you find it is acceptable to take care of yourself. In the process others will learn how to take care of their needs just by being around you. Employing the affirmation, "I have love and compassion for myself," while tapping gently on the H9 point of the heart meridian, (the inner aspect of the fifth digit of the left hand where the skin meets the nail), you will have learned the important skill of bringing yourself back into the present moment. While in the present moment you cannot worry about what you think might be lacking in the future. Your ability to generate loving kindness calms and settles those around you as everyone senses an enhanced state of well-being.

You have discovered that being present is the greatest goal of your efforts. In identifying unexplored anger and fear you refuse to take refuge in fight or flight. You are now capable of standing your ground and living first hand, unfiltered, experience. You are now able to stop struggling, acknowledge your own ignorance, and learn something new from each thought and emotion you have. No longer in need of external excitement to keep interested a new blanket of peace surrounds you. Your appreciation for life increases many fold. Your energy increases, your relationships improve, your efforts are more effective, and you get sick less since your immune system has less internal stress to deal with.

By identifying destructive self-talk and affirming that you will remain in the moment, though difficulties continue to plague you, you give yourself the gift of empowerment. As you relax and calm the monkey mind within, the roots of your struggles are unearthed. Once these harmful thoughts, efforts, and actions are replaced, conditions are ripe for peace, harmony, presence, compassion, and hope to flourish. You have given in to the moment. Surrender and acceptance are your friends. You have discovered the person behind the mask and are waiting to learn more with the next breath.

In time you will discover that meditation offers the vehicle that allows you to sit and watch your inner world. Your willingness to accept this gift opens the way to a life of greater clarity, trust, intention, and peace. You possess the keys to your own healing. In using these keys you make it possible for others to heal their deepest wounds also.

Notes

SECTION ONE

Chapter Two - WHOSE TIMETABLE ARE YOU ON?

[1]Carlson, Richard & Joseph Bailey. *Slowing Down to the Speed of Life: How to Create a More Peaceful Life from the Inside Out.* San Francisco: Harper, 1997, 94

SECTION TWO

Chapter Three - DISCOVERING NEW SOURCES OF ENERGY

[1]Nisenbaum R, Reyes M, Unger ER, Reeves WC. "Factor analysis of symptoms among subjects with unexplained chronic fatigue: what can we learn about chronic fatigue syndrome?" (*Journal of Psychosomatic Research* 56),171-178, 2004

[2]Sherwood, Keith, *Chakra Therapy For Personal Growth and Healing* (St. Paul: Llewellyn, 2001).

[3]Diemer, Deedre. *The ABC's of Chakra Therapy: A Workbook* (York Beach, ME: Weiser, 1998) pp38-73.

[4]Teeguarden, Iona Marsaa. *A Complete Guide to Acupressure* (Tokyo: Japan Publications, 1996), p. 106.

[5]Davies, Clair. *The Trigger Point Therapy Workbook: Your Self-Treatment Guide For Pain Relief* (Oakland: New Harbinger Publications, 2001).

[6]Kabat-Zinn. *Full Catastrophe Living: Using the Wisdom of Your Body and Mind to Face Stress, Pain and Illness* (New York: Dell 1990), pp 75-93.

Chapter Four. SEARCHING FOR GOLD AND FINDING IT

[1]"The Gold Rush." http\\www.pbs.org\goldrush\discovery\html

[2]Garofalo, J.P., " Perceived Optimism and Chronic Pain" In *Personality Characteristics of Patients With Pain* R. J. Gatchel & J. N. Weisberg, eds. (Washington, D.C.: American Psychological Association, 2000), p. 208.

Chapter Five. FIRE PLUS O_2 → A NEW YOU

[1]Wangyal, Tenzin Rinpoche. *The Tibetan Yogas of Dream and Sleep* (New York: Snow Lion Publications, 1998) p.26

[2]Hathaway, S.R., McKinley, J.C. (1943). *The Minnesota Multiphasic Personality schedule (revised).* (Minneapolis: University of Minnesota Press, 1943).

[3]Deardorff, W.W. (2000). "The MMPI-2 and Chronic Pain" in *Personality Characteristics of Patients With Pain* edited by R.J. Gatchel & J.N. Weisberg (Washington, D.C.: American Psychological Association, 2000) pp. 109-125.

[4]Martin, P. *The Zen Path through Depression* (San Francisco: Harper, 1999) p. 11.

[5]Satchidananda, Sri Swami, *The Yoga Sutras of Patanjali* (Yogaville, Virginia: Integral Yoga Publications, 1999), p. 125.

SECTION THREE

INTRODUCTION

[1]Kant, Immanuel, "Groundwork of the Metaphysic of Morals" In de Botton, A. *Status Anxiety* (New York: Pantheon Books, 2004), p. 99.

Chapter Six. MORE THAN A PHYSICAL BODY: CAN YOU FEEL IT?

[1]DeGood, Douglas, E. "Relationship of Pain-Coping Strategies To Adjustment and Functioning" In *Personality Characteristics of Patients With Pain* edited by R.J. Gatchel & J.N. Weisberg (Washington, D.C.: American Psychological Association, 2000), pp. 147-148.

[2]Devi, Nischala Joy. *The Healing Path of Yoga: Time-Honored Wisdom and Scientifically Proven Methods that Alleviate Stress, Open Your Heart, and Enrich Your Life* (New York: Three Rivers Press, 2000) pp. 68-79.

[3]Sherwood, Keith. *Chakra Therapy for Personal Growth and Healing* (St. Paul: Llewellyn Publications, 2001), p145-147.

[4]Ruiz, Don, M. *The Four Agreements.* (San Rafeal: Amber-Allen, 1997), pp. 25-46.

[5]The DREAMS Foundation, http://www.dreams.ca/dreams.htm.

[6]Tenzin Wangyal Rinpoche. *The Tibetan Yogas Of Dream And Sleep.* (Ithica, New York: Snow Lion, 1998), p. 23.

[7]E. S. Peterson, ed., *Light And Liberty: Reflections on the Pursuit of Happiness.* (New York: The Modern Library, 2004), p. 11.

[8]Chodron, Pema. *Start Where You Are: A Guide to Compassionate Living.* (Boston: Shambhala, 2001).

Chapter Eight. EFFORT

[1]Levine, Stephen. *A Year to Live* (New York: Bell Tower, 1997).

[2]Hanh, Thich Nhat. *The Heart of the Buddha's Teaching: Transforming Suffering into Peace, Joy, and Liberation* (New York: Broadway Books, 1998), pp. 49-118.

[3]The Dalai Lama., Cutler, H.C. *The Art of Happiness At Work* (New York: Riverhead Books, 2003), pp. 49-66.

[4]Nichols, M.P. *The Lost Art of Listening: How Learning to Listen Can Improve Relationships* (New York: Guilford Press, 1995), p. 112.

[5]Suzuki, Shunryu. *Zen Mind, Beginner's Mind.* (New York: Weatherhill, 1997).

SECTION FOUR

INTRODUCTION

[1]Calhoun, J. B. "Population Density and Social Pathology" (Scientific American 206, 1962) 139-148.

[2]Obsessive-Compulsive Foundation. "What is OCD?" (http://www.ocfoundation.org).

[3]Chodron, P. Start *When You Are: A Guide to Compassionate Living.* (Boston: Shambhala, 1994).

Chapter Nine. DEEPER MEDITATION

[1]De Botton, A. *Status Anxiety.* (New York: Pantheon, 2004), p. 194.

[2]Glass, J. "Ingredients of Love," (*Ascent* 24, Winter2004), pp. 13-17.

[3]Salzberg, S. Loving-Kindness: *The Revolutionary Art of Happiness.* (Boston: Shambhala, 1995).

[4]Chodron, P., *Start Where You Are: A Guide to Compassionate Living.* (Boston: Shambhala, 2001), pp. 33-43.

[5]Treder, M. "The Incipient Posthuman" (http//www.incipientposthuman.com, 2004).

Chapter Ten. TIME FOR HEALING

[1]"Discipline at Home", *Spanking: Facts and Fiction* (EPOCH – USA, http://www.stophitting.com)

[2]Kabat-Zinn, J. *Wherever You Go There You Are: Mindfulness Meditation in Everyday Life.* (New York: Hyperion, 1994).

SECTION FIVE

INTRODUCTION

[1]"Meditation XVII: No Man is an island" (from: *Devotions Upon Emergent Occasions*, 1624, http://isu.indstate.edu/ilnprof/ENG451/ISLAND)

Chapter Eleven. LOOKING TO OTHERS

[1]Trungpa, Chogyam. *The Myth of Freedom and the Way of Meditation*, (Boston: Shambhala, 2002) pp. 51-59.

[2]Herrigel, Eugen. *The Method of Zen.* (New York: Vintage Books, 1974) pp. 123-125.

Chapter Twelve. THE PATH TO HEALTH IS PAVED WITH INTENTION

[1]Hallowell, E.M. M.D. *The Childhood Roots of Adult Happiness.* (New York: Ballantine. 2002) pp. 103-123.

[2]Ibid.

Bibliography

Birx, Ellen. *Healing Zen*. New York, Viking Compass, 2002.

Calhoun, J. B. "Population Density and Social Pathology." *Scientific American* 206 (1962): 139-148.

CancerWise. "Impact of Expressive Writing on Cancer." April 2002, http://www.cancerwise.org/April_2002/print.cfm?id=239B5B3C-7FF1-4AEE-B919EC54D7F79F16&method=DisplayFull

Carlson, Richard & Joseph Bailey. *Slowing Down to the Speed of Life: How to Create a More Peaceful Life from the Inside Out*, Harper, San Francisco: Harper, 1997.

Chodron, Pema. *The Places that Scare You: A Guide to Fearlessness in Difficult Times*. Boston: Shambhala, 2001.

Chodron, Pema. *Start Where You Are: A Guide to Compassionate Living*. Boston: Shambhala, 1994, 2001.

Davies, Clair. *The Trigger Point Therapy Workbook: Your Self-Treatment Guide For Pain Relief*. Oakland: New Harbinger Publications, 2001

Deardorff, W.W. "The MMPI-2 and Chronic Pain." In *Personality Characteristics of Patients With Pain*, edited by R.J. Gatchel & J.N. Weisberg. Washington, D.C.: American Psychological Association, 2000.

De Botton, A. *Status Anxiety*. New York: Pantheon, 2004.

DeGood, Douglas, E. Relationship of Pain-Coping Strategies To Adjustment and Functioning. In *Personality Characteristics of Patients With Pain*, edited by R.J. Gatchel & J.N. Weisberg. Washington, D.C.: American Psychological Association, 2000.

Devi, Nischala Joy. *The Healing Path of Yoga: Time-Honored Wisdom and Scientifically Proven Methods that Alleviate Stress, Open Your Heart, and Enrich Your Life*. New York: Three Rivers Press, 2000.

Diemer, Deedre. *The ABC's of Chakra Therapy: A Workbook*. York Beach, ME: Weiser, 1998.

EPOCH–USA. "Discipline at Home. Spanking: Facts and Fiction." The Center For Effective Discipline. http://www.stophitting.com

Freeman, Richard. *Yoga Breathing. Sounds*. Boulder, CO: True, 2002.

Garofalo, J.P. (2000). "Perceived Optimism and Chronic Pain." In *Personality Characteristics of Patients With Pain*, edited byR.J. Gatchel & J.N. Weisberg. Washington, D.C.: American Psychological Association, 2000.Glass, J. "Ingredients of Love," Ascent 24 (Winter2004): 13-17.

Glass, J. "Ingredients of Love," *Ascent* 24 (Winter2004): 13-17.

Goldberg, Natalie & Dosho Port. *Zen Howl: Revealing this One Great Life. Sounds.* Boulder, CO: True, 2003.

Hallowell, E.M. M.D. *The Childhood Roots of Adult Happiness.* New York: Ballantine, 2002.

Hanh, Thich Nhat. *The Heart of the Buddha's Teaching: Transforming Suffering into Peace, Joy, and Liberation.* New York: Broadway Books, 1998.

Hanh, Thich Nhat. *Anger: Wisdom for Cooling the Flames.* New York: Penguin,2001.

Hathaway, S.R., McKinley, J.C. *The Minnesota Multiphasic Personality schedule (revised).* Minneapolis: University of Minnesota Press, 1943.

Herrigel, Eugen. *The Method of Zen.* New York: Vintage Books, 1974.

Hyman Mark. "Practicing Medicine for the Future". *Alternative Therapies in Health and Medicine*, Vol. 10, No. 4.(July/August 2004): 83-89.

Indiana State University Trustees. "Meditation XVII: No Man is an island" from Donne, John, *Devotions Upon Emergent Occasions.* 1624. http://isu.indstate.edu/ilnprof/ENG451/ISLAND

Kabat-Zinn, J. *Full Catastrophe Living: Using the Wisdom of Your Body and Mind to Face Stress, Pain, and Illness.* New York: Dell, 1990.

Kabat-Zinn, J. *Wherever You Go There You Are: Mindfulness Meditation in Everyday Life.* New York: Hyperion, 1994.

Kant, Immanuel. "Groundwork of the Metaphysic of Morals." In de Botton, A. *Status Anxiety.* New York: Pantheon Books, 2004.

Levine, Stephen. *A Year to Live: How to Life this Year as If It Were Your Last.* New York: Bell Tower, 1997.

Martin, P. *The Zen Path through Depression.* San Francisco: Harper, 1999.

Piper, Watty. *The Little Engine that Could.* New York: Penguin,1976.

Mind Tools Ltd. Morgan, Michael. *Creating Workforce Innovations.* A concise explanation of the Reframing Matrix- Looking at problems with a different perspective. http://mindtools.com/pages/article/newCT_05.htm

Nichols, M.P. *The Lost Art of Listening: How Learning to Listen Can Improve Relationships.* New York: Guilford Press, 1995.

Nisenbaum R, Reyes M, Unger ER, Reeves WC. "Factor analysis of symptoms among subjects with unexplained chronic fatigue: what can we learn about chronic fatigue syndrome?" *Journal of Psychosomatic Research* 56 (2004):171-178.

Obsessive-Compulsive Foundation. "What is OCD?" http://www.ocfoundation.org.

Peterson, E. S., *Light And Liberty: Reflections on the Pursuit of Happiness,* ed. New York: The Modern Library, 2004.

Pink, Arthur. *The Fear of the Lord is the Beginning of Wisdom. Proverbs 1:7.* http://www.pbministries.org/books/pink/Miscellaneous/fear_of_the_lord.htm.

Rinpoche, Tenzin Wangyal. *The Tibetan Yogas Of Dream And Sleep*. Ithaca, New York: Snow Lion, 1998.

Ruiz, Don, M. *The Four Agreements*. San Rafael: Amber-Allen, 1997. http://www.dreams.ca/dreams.htm. The DREAMS Foundation.

Salzberg, S. *Loving-Kindness: The Revolutionary Art of Happiness*. Boston: Shambhala, 1995.

Satchidananda, Sri Swami. *The Yoga Sutras of Patanjali*. Yogaville, Virginis: Integral Yoga Publications, 1999.

Sherwood, Keith. *Chakra Therapy for Personal Growth and Healing*. St. Paul: Llewellyn Publications, 2001.

Sutton, John. *Memory,* The Stanford Encyclopedia of Philosophy, http:www.scence.uva.nl/?seop/archives/spr2003/entries/memory/

Suzuki, Shunryu. *Zen Mind, Beginner's Mind Weatherhill*, New York: 1997.

The Dalai Lama., H. C. Cutler. *The Art of Happiness At Work*. New York: Riverhead Books, 2003.

The DREAMS Foundation. http://www.dreams.ca/dreams.htm.

The Gold Rush. http\\www.pbs.org\goldrush\discovery\html

Treder, M. "The Incipient Posthuman." http//www.incipientposthuman.com. 2004.

Teeguarden, Iona Marsaa. *A Complete Guide to Acupressure*. Tokyo: Japan Publications, 1996.

"Scientists Study the Impact of Expressive Writing on Cancer." *CancerWise* (April, 2002) University of Texas M.D. Anderson Cancer Center. http://www.cancer-wise.org/april_2002/display.cfm?id=239B5B3C-7FF1-4AEE-B919EC54D7F79F16&method=displayFull&color=green

The Gold Rush. http\\www.pbs.org\goldrush\discovery\html

Trungpa, Chogyam. *The Myth of Freedom and the Way of Meditation*. Boston: Shambhala, 2002.

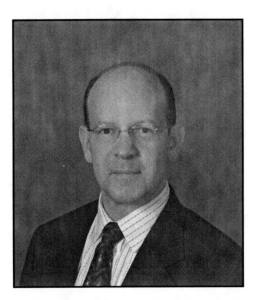

JOHN J. INZERILLO, a practicing medical oncologist for over fifteen years, has offered many patients cutting-edge therapies through cooperative oncology groups sponsored by the National Cancer Institute. Through his participation in clinical trials, he has contributed to the clinical data base on the treatment of such cancers as breast, colon, lung, prostate, lymphoma, and leukemia.

In the treatment and management of cancer Doctor Inzerillo is receptive to the use of complementary therapies such as mindfulness training, yoga, meditation, and prayer. As a result of his ten years of meditation and yoga training he has developed techniques that facilitate personal balance and help bring mental and physical restoration to the workplace, home environment, and interpersonal encounters. In the clinical arena, he has written mentoring articles for medical students stressing the importance of presence and compassion while caring for those in need.

Volunteering his time as a restorative yoga instructor for his patients and their caregivers has been a privilege for Doctor Inzerillo. He successfully guides them though the challenges of anxiety, depression, frustration, and pain associated with illness. He balances these efforts and energies by enjoying time with his wife and two sons.

www.johninzerillo.com
www.passionbeyondpain.com

OTHER WELLNESS BOOKS
FROM HUMANICS

Body, Self & Soul - Sustaining Integration by Jack Lee Rosenberg, Ph.D. & Marjorie Rand, Ph.D. with Diana Asay

Inner Bridges - a Guide to Energy Movement and Body Structure by Fredrick Smith, M.D.

The Tao of Calm - 81 Meditations for Everyday Living by Pamela Metz

The Tao of Recovery - A Quiet Path to Wellness by Jim McGregor

While You Are Expecting - Your Own Prenatal Classroom by F. Rene Van De Carr, M.D. & Marc Lehrer, Ph.D.

Humanics Publishing Group

www.humanicspub.com

Order Form

Bill To: _____

Ship To: _____

_____ _____

_____ _____

_____ _____

Tel: _____ Fax: _____   Tel: _____ Fax: _____

Email Address: _____   Email Address: _____

METHOD OF PAYMENT

☐ Bill Me ☐ MasterCard ☐ Discover
☐ Check Enclosed ☐ VISA ☐ American Express   Card Number _____   Exp. Date ___ Signature ___

ISBN	TITLE	PRICE	QUANTITY	TOTAL

ORDERING INFORMATION

Call Toll Free **1.800.874.8844** to place orders via credit card or to bill orders to your account. (International customers call +1.561.533.6231)

Mail orders to: **Humanics Publishing Group, 12 S. Dixie Hwy., Ste. 203, Lake Worth, FL 33460 USA**

Fax Orders Toll Free to **1.888.874.8844**, 24 hours a day, 7 days a week. (International customers fax to +1.561.533.6233)
Please allow 7-10 days for delivery.

SHIPPING/HANDLING
For orders under $100.00 net,
S&H charges will be as follows:
$10.00 for the first book, and
$2.00 for each additional book.
For orders over $100.00 net,
S&H charges will be 15% of Net.

SHIPPING/HANDLING

TOTAL